PASSPORT
to
Pleasure

PASSPORT
to
Pleasure

*The Hottest Sex
from Around the World*

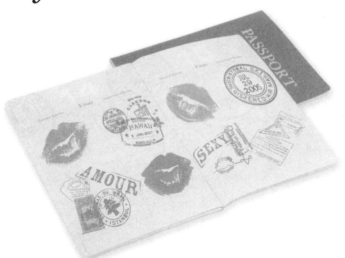

LAURA CORN

S|S|E

SIMON SPOTLIGHT ENTERTAINMENT

New York   London   Toronto   Sydney

AN IMPORTANT NOTE TO READERS

This book contains the opinions and ideas of its author. It is intended to provide helpful and informative material on the subjects addressed in the publication, and it is intended solely for the use of informed, consenting, and hopefully monogamous adults who want to rejuvenate, enliven, and sustain a great sexual relationship. This book is sold with the understanding that the author is not a medical doctor or therapist, and that neither the authors nor the publisher is engaged in rendering medical, health, therapeutic, or any other kind of personal professional services in this book.

The reader is cautioned that following the suggestions and scenarios herein is strictly voluntary and at the reader's own risk and discretion. Every individual is unique; therefore, you should not employ any position or products that is not suitable to your physical or sexual limitations Also, this book contains suggestions of sex acts that may be illegal in some jurisdictions. You should know your local laws about sex before engaging in any activity.

The author and publisher do not sponsor and are not affiliated with nor responsible for any product or third-party website or resource material referenced in this book. The author and publisher specifically disclaim all responsibility for any liability, loss or risk, personal or otherwise, which is incurred as a consequence, directly or indirectly, of the use and application of any of the content of this book.

S|S|E

Simon Spotlight Entertainment
A Division of Simon & Schuster, Inc.
1230 Avenue of the Americas
New York, NY 10020

Copyright © 2008 by Laura Corn

First Simon Spotlight Entertainment trade paperback edition December 2008

SIMON SPOTLIGHT ENTERTAINMENT and colophon are trademarks of Simon & Schuster, Inc.

For information about special discounts for bulk purchases, please contact Simon & Schuster Special Sales at 1-800-456-6798 or business@simonandschuster.com.

Designed by Lucky Colchester

Manufactured in the United States of America

10 9 8 7 6 5 4 3 2 1

Library of Congress Cataloging-in-Publication Data is available.

ISBN-13: 978-1-4169-6404-9
ISBN-10:   1-4169-6404-5

*This book is dedicated to
couples everywhere who believe that nothing
spices up a relationship like new experiences.*

Acknowledgments

I feel blessed to have had so many talented people work on this book. Thank you to everyone who has taken this journey around the world with me.

To Jeff: You are the love of my life and the greatest lover in the world. Your passion for travel and adventure has opened my eyes to romantic, erotic, naughty nights, international style.

To Stacie Harb: Your brilliant creativity and enthusiasm has guided this book from its conception to its completion. Thank you for being my True North.

To Marty Bishop: I've said it before: You are the most talented writer I know. This book would not have been possible without your humor, style, and insight. If I had a ship, the figurehead would be you.

To Mads: Is there anything you don't do well? My gosh, girl, the cultural sex secrets you came up with curled my toes. Here's hoping they curl a million more.

To the great literary agent Frank Weiman: Thank you for finding me the best home possible with Simon and Schuster. I look forward to more adventures together.

To Edward: There would be no stamps on my passport without you. This book would not have been a reality without your excitement, enthusiasm and encouragement. Truly, I owe this book—and volumes of gratitude—to you.

To my wonderful team at Simon and Schuster:

To Cara Bedick: My editor extraordinaire, thank you for your tireless work, patience, and invaluable guidance on this trek.

To Jennifer Bergstrom: For believing in me and in this project, and for helping to get it off the ground, I thank you.

To Michael Nagin: I don't just like the book cover; I love it! Thank you for doing what no one thought could be done—You made us all happy, and you did it with style.

A special thanks to My Smart and Sexy International Research Team: Madeline Glass, Jina Bacarr, Eden Bradley, Rachel Kramer Bussel, Patricia Cihodaru, Py Kim Conant, Miss Dirty Martini, Achsa Vissel, Lisa Wixon, and Kristina Wright. Ladies, thank you, one and all.

To Lauren Kutasi: The talented illustrator whose sexy images are peppered throughout this book. Thank you.

Contents

Introduction

Laura Takes a Trip

This whole project started, oddly enough, as a vacation. After more than ten years of writing, I decided it was time to relax and see a bit of the world. Jeff and I went to Europe for our first stop, and it was everything we'd hoped for—beautiful, relaxing, and romantic. (We got to go roller-skating through the streets of Paris! What a delicious memory, right up to the part where I tumbled and ended up in a wrist brace for the rest of my trip. Ouch.)

Travel is always an eye-opening experience, and I expected to learn lots of new things. I just didn't expect to learn new things about *seduction*.

Over the years, I've written hundreds of seductions for couples looking to build a better relationship. Some of these seductions focused on romance, some explored hotter sex, some were designed to improve communication and intimacy. But all the seductions in my books had one big thing in common. They were created to solve the one universal concern all couples eventually face: *predictability*.

If you've ever found yourself in that kind of rut, then you're in good company, because it happens to almost all couples at some time. The solution, of course, is to put the fun and romance, and the intimacy back at the top of your to-do list. I've spent my previous seven books helping readers kick-start that process with hundreds of ways. In fact, I was beginning to think I might have discovered *all* the ways one lover could surprise another, and that's why I was ready for a vacation.

But while traveling, I began to realize just how clever people are when it comes to sex. The men and women of France, Italy—and England, and everywhere we visited—had found ways to add spice to their relationships, but they were often *different* ways, unique to their part of the world. Some of these sexy practices sprang from local culture, some seemed to be accidents of history, and many were just fun bedroom tricks I had never heard of. My cool vacation suddenly got a lot more interesting. "*Really? You do* what *over here? Tell me more!*" Eventually, my new hobby grew into a research project. Jeff, as usual, got to be my study partner and experimental subject as we explored the *dormitorios, cameras, shinshitsu, спальня, chambres à coucher*, and bedrooms of the world.

Seduction Around the World

In love and in writing, you never know where inspiration will come from. As usual, some of these seductions are based on stories from men and women I've talked to, and for this book I went even further. When you start looking for it, you'll find great sex *everywhere*: in history books, scholarly reports, museums, travel guides, websites, surveys, and books. I've linked each seduction in *Passport to Pleasure* with the city or country that inspired me to write about it. That doesn't mean this is the only place on Earth where couples use a particular technique, but it probably means they are famous for it, or proud of it. Some seductions are "cultural cocktails"—based on fun ideas from several countries. I didn't choose specific tricks because they were foreign—several of them are from America, in fact—but because they were interesting, surprising, and above all, arousing. You'll probably also learn a thing or two about different cultures around the world, which I hope you'll enjoy that as much as I did, but that's really just a happy side effect. In the end, you'll follow these seductions because they show you how to have a stronger, more intimate relationship . . . and to have some crazy fun doing it.

The Power of Anticipation

Every week, you or your partner will flip through the seductions, choose one, and tear it out of the book, along the perforations. And at that moment, you're invoking one of the most powerful forces in the world: *anticipation*. When you rip open that page, you're making a promise, a commitment to make something wonderful happen, and your sweetie will spend the next several days wondering what kind of surprise you're planning. To make sure it remains a mystery, each seduction is folded over and sealed shut, like an envelope. Your lover can't read ahead and spoil the surprise.

So if the seductions are sealed, how do you know which one to pick? There are clues printed on the outside. Each one is marked *For HER Eyes Only,* or *For HIS Eyes Only,* and there are icons that can help you plan for weather, transportation, and expense. If you start reading your seduction—in private, of course—and decide that you can't make that one work for some reason, rip out a different one. *Just don't let it slide.* Your partner is expecting something. And you'll both enjoy that growing sense of anticipation all week long.

Building a Better Relationship

On the surface, it couldn't be easier. You just do what the seductions say, and have the greatest date of your life. A week later, your lover does the same for you. But on a deeper level, here's what's really happening: *you're both learning*. I don't just mean sex tricks, though there are a *lot* of those in these pages. You're both going to be developing better relationship habits—basic, thoughtful, respectful, romantic habits, the kind of things men and women too often forget to do after a while. But these skills aren't presented as lessons in this book. They're not things you have to study. Instead, they're simply built right into the seductions. You do them without even thinking about them, while you're having fun. And then, because they work, you find yourself instinctively doing them more often. Before you know it, they're part of you, and each of you becomes a better partner to the other.

Props

Lots of these seductions encourage you to buy extra little items to dress up the event. Most are inexpensive and easy to find, and to help you locate any that aren't available in your town, I've included a list of websites and mail-order catalogs in the back of the book. Don't just ignore these special ingredients! It's extra touches like these that convince your sweetheart that you really mean it. If you can't find what I've suggested, *substitute*. Use your imagination. It really is the effort that counts.

Take a Little Trip

Let *Passport to Pleasure* take you on an unforgettable trip. This is a year's worth of weekly seductions. Open each envelope to find out what's hot in the country that inspired this seduction—its sexy music and books, or perhaps its famous seducers, its most popular sex toy and sexiest lingerie, and that country's traditional tools of seduction, as well as sexy facts and stats. Did you know that South Koreans have more sex per week than couples anywhere else in the world? Get inspired!

Quick Start Guide

Icons

There are symbols on the cover of each sealed page to help you decide which Seduction to choose.

 You're going outside. Save for warm weather.

 You'll need a car. (Clean out the backseat!)

 Could mean you're preparing a meal, a treat, or going out to eat.

$ Indicates the anticipated cost of everything you need to purchase for a particular Seduction, like meals, lingerie, or gifts. These figures *don't* include items you already have, like a phone, car, email address, or bedroom toy. Most Seductions are quite affordable. Only a very few cost more than one hundred dollars, and you may save those for special occasions like birthdays or anniversaries.

> No $ at all means it's free or under $10.
> $ means $10–$25.
> $$ means $30–$60.
> $$$ means $65–$100.
> $$$$ means more than $100.

 Special Seduction:
one for a Birthday,

 one for a special day,

 one for a very special day.

Pick a time, tear out a page

This is the most fun part of *Passport to Pleasure!* (Right after the, um, sex.) Commit to a regular time to get together with your partner and look through the book. Most readers say that Sunday evening works best. Talk about the titles, and consider the icons. Each of you will remove a Seduction from the book, tearing along the perforations. Because they are folded over and closed, neither of you will know what the other is planning. *But each of you has now made a promise to seduce the other.* Open your sealed Seduction, read it alone, and then start planning your sexy surprises.

Anticipation

You may be instructed to do something special to get your mate's attention, hours or days before you finish the Seduction. Don't skip them! They are designed to create a sense of anticipation. They keep your lover focused on *you* throughout the week. They are, in short, a form of foreplay.

Dress It Up

Turn an ordinary come-on into irresistible foreplay. Special outfits, lights, music, meals, etc. can be scaled to suit your budget or match your imagination. But don't pass them up. They're fun now—and will stir up spectacular memories in the future.

Good Vibrations

Not all couples use bedroom toys, but those who do find that they add an extra dimension of fun to foreplay. A handful of Seductions involve the mutual use of toys, and if you don't have any yet, this is a perfect opportunity to see what the buzz is about. Check the Specialty Shops page for some recommended vendors.

Go with the Flow

Your lover is going to spring some surprises on you! Some may seem silly at first, or oddly out of character. But go along with it. You're going to love it. (And you're going to want your partner to play along with *you* when it's your turn.)

Laura Corn, I just can't do that!

Yes, you can. Sooner or later, especially if you're a shy person, chances are you'll come across a Seduction that seems too wild or too extravagant or simply too much for you. I say—just do it! Do it, do it, do it! Your partner will be thrilled.

I mean, really, <u>no way!</u>

Oh, you mean you don't have a car, or a yard, or some essential ingredient specified in the Seduction? Well, okay. Skip it. Pick a different one. There are plenty to choose from.

Hygiene

Your mate is going to be coming on to you. Sometimes you will have no warning at all. But a sexy Seduction (and even an entire relationship) can be short-circuited by poor hygiene. Clean hair, clean skin, clean teeth, fresh breath: That's the uniform we put on to play the game of love. Suit up!

The magic number

There are 26 Seductions for men, marked *For HIS Eyes Only*, and 26 seductions for women, marked *For HER Eyes Only*.

It will take some time to get there, though. Here's the math: if you and your partner alternate tearing out a sealed Seduction each week, this book will last for almost one entire year. That is an ambitious schedule, not to mention an incredible workout program. That's a whole year of new erotic tricks, exhilarating challenges, intimate moments, and breathtaking orgasms. Name one other product that offers as much bang for the buck. Seriously. We should raise the price.

It all starts the moment you begin ripping out pages. So go ahead—take a little trip . . .

PASSPORT
to
Pleasure

seduction no. 1

Never Out of Style

POLAND

FOR *his* EYES ONLY

 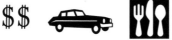

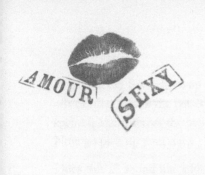

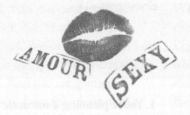
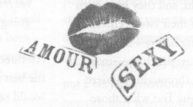

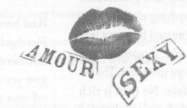
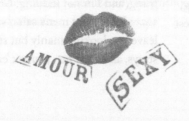

seduction no. 2

Pop It Like It's Hot

USA

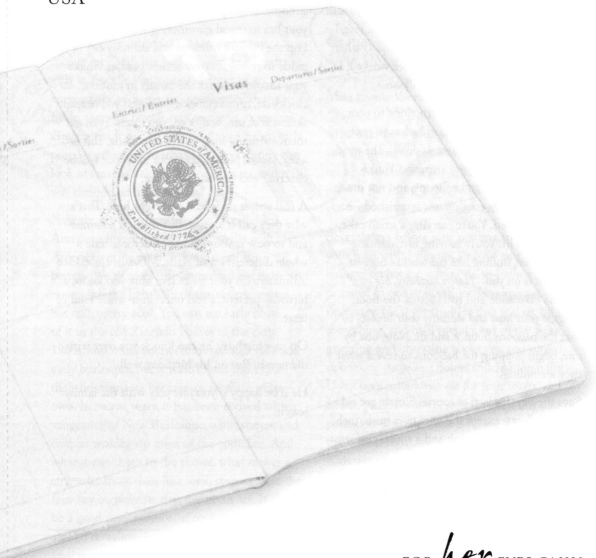

FOR *her* EYES ONLY

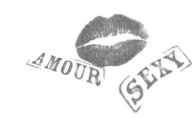
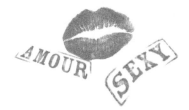
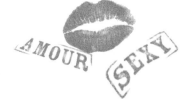

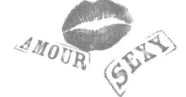

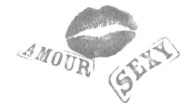

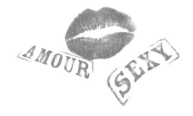
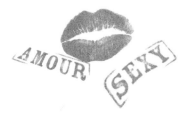

seduction no. **3**

The Tiny Mailman

MOUNTAIN VIEW, CALIFORNIA, USA

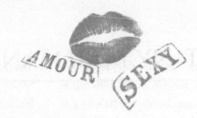

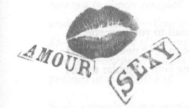

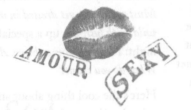
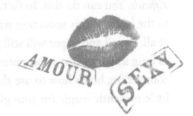
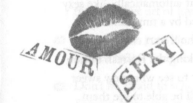
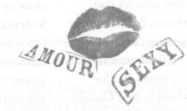
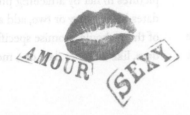
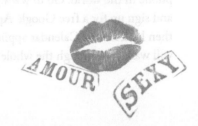

seduction no. 4

Fantasy Box

CULTURAL COCKTAIL: FRANCE, SPAIN, GERMANY

FOR *his* EYES ONLY

$

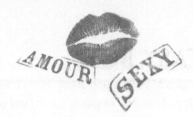
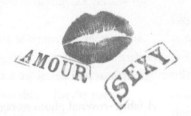

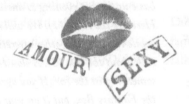
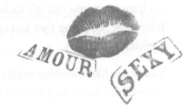
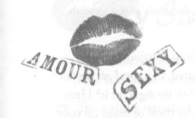
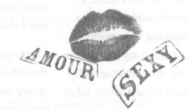
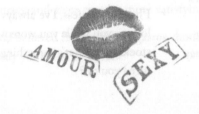
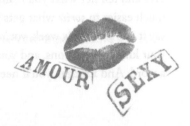

seduction no. 5

Honeylingus

BEIJING, CHINA

FOR *his* EYES ONLY

Be sure to set a romantic scene for her, with candles in the bathroom and music on the stereo. Oh, and one more thing. Get an old washable blanket and lay it across your bed. Trust me on this; she'll be much more relaxed with your next move if she knows she won't have to clean up a big mess afterward.

As she finishes her bath, bring her the honey and offer her a proposition. *"I want to play a little game with you. After I leave the bathroom, I want you to hide six dabs of honey anywhere on your body. Anywhere at all,"* you say, *"kind of like this."* Squeeze a few drops on the side of her neck, just above her collarbone. Don't let it run; instead, rub it with your fingertip into a small, sticky circle.

"And then," you continue, *"I'm going to try to find them all. Like this."* Lean in and lick it off. No, *suck* it off, and nibble it off, and just in case you missed some, move up to her ear, and the back of her neck, gently nuzzling and kissing her everywhere you go. Make it perfectly clear that you expect to give your tongue a real workout tonight. *"Remember, six little dabs. Hide them anywhere, front and back, and then come join me in the bedroom."*

Find your honey's honey. Connect the dots with your tongue. Work the areas that don't usually get enough attention. Knees and toes, shoulders and wrists—they all deserve your loving and licking. Breasts, nipples, thighs, bum—pay them all a visit. Finally, of course, you need to focus on your real goal, your honeypie's honeypot. At this point, you should take your cue from my new bar friend, the one with the amazing China tale: Every story needs a *dàtuányuán*. A happy ending!

美满结局

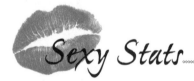

Sexy Stats

- Honey has been associated with sensuality for millennia. It is written about in classic texts such as the *Perfumed Garden*, the *Kama Sutra*, and the Bible, and almost always speaks to love, richness, and beauty.

- Honey is considered an aphrodisiac. This may be because honey is easily digested, and its sugar quickly converts to energy. Looking for a fast way to refuel? Nutritionists say two tablespoons of honey and two 400 IUs of vitamin E will give you roughly four hours of energy.

- Honey Dust is the most popular item in the extensive Kama Sutra line of sensual products. It's real honey—prized as a skin conditioner in India—in powder form in different fruit flavors.

- In the film *9 1/2 Weeks*, John asks Elizabeth to stick out her tongue and then squeezes honey onto it. It's one scene that will definitely whet your appetite for honey-flavored skin.

No. 5 HONEYLINGUS

INGREDIENTS

1 quart of milk
1 clean girl
1 blanket, washable, to protect your bedsheets
(big towel will do, if she's tiny; giant latex
sheet, if she's kinky)

1 squeezable bottle of honey
1 strong tongue

I COULD HARDLY BELIEVE MY LUCK. A girlfriend and I were sitting in the bar of a beautiful restaurant in LA when, through a string of conversational coincidences, I found myself face-to-face with a famous rock star. I might have been a tiny bit starstruck. I used to save my allowance to buy his cassettes, and here he is, talking to me. Cool.

I didn't learn anything about him that you couldn't read for yourself on Wikipedia, though. Darn it. Ah, but his *friend*—now here was a guy who had a fascinating tale to tell. He wasn't quite as famous, but he was certainly very rich and devilishly handsome. The buzz on the rock star's friend was that he had lived a bachelor's dream and had been with thousands of women around the world.

I couldn't help myself. I just had to ask. I know this is not your normal polite conversation, but hey, I write sex books for a living, so I jumped right to the big question. "What would you say is the best sex you've ever had?"

He didn't even blink. Without hesitation, he answered, "The Milk and Honey Massage, in Beijing, China." His eyes twinkled as he went on to describe the most erotic massage technique I have ever heard of. It involved milk and honey, slathered on with a soft brush, and then lovingly removed with a long, slow and exceedingly thorough tongue bath. By the time he finished his story I was breathing hard and more than a little aroused. Wow. I wanted my *own* Milk and Honey Massage!

I knew my readers would want one, too, so I took the idea home and started to work it out. After a few weeks of blissful experimentation, I finally had a recipe that any man can follow. Yes, it involves milk and honey, but at its core, this technique is about *attention*. Complete, total focus on your partner's sensual pleasure. It's pampering. Indulgence. Sexual service + romance + a killer skin-conditioning treatment = every woman's dream! (And it costs practically nothing. Seriously, dollars to orgasms, it's the best value in the book. No need to mention that to your sweetie.)

The ingredients might already be in your own home, and if not, it's easy to find a quart of milk and a small squeeze jar of honey. Tie them together with a ribbon or string, and attach a note to them in the fridge: *Don't touch! I have a surprise for you this week!*

Now you've got her. Promise her a surprise, create some romantic anticipation, and you're halfway to Grrreat Sex already. Pick a night when you're staying in and offer to draw a bath for her. Add three or four cups of milk to create a special treat, an *exfoliant milk bath*. (Yes, there's some actual science at work here. Ever see those ads for skin products that contain alpha hydroxy acids? Milk has one of those.)

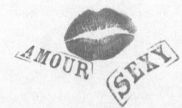

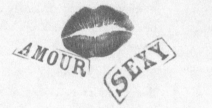
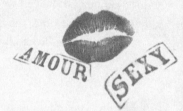
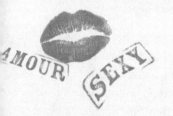

seduction no. 6

Satin Strokes

CULTURAL COCKTAIL: THAILAND, USA

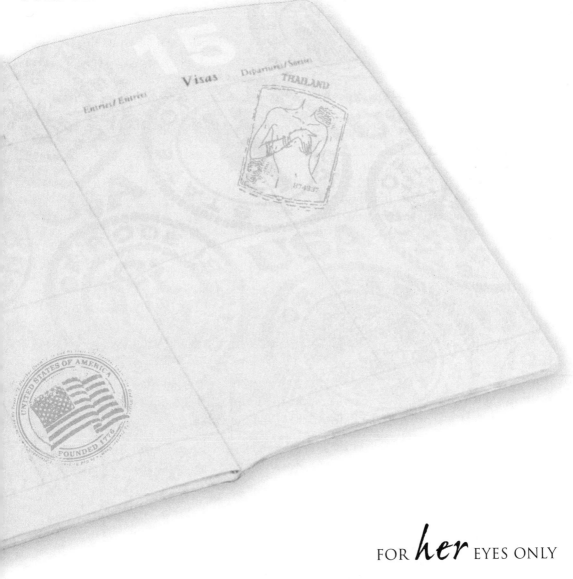

FOR *her* EYES ONLY

$

arms under his and stroke his hardening shaft, *"Look at us."* Your satiny fingers on his erection and the slickness of your slip will surround him, and your whispered reminders to watch what's happening in the mirror will make him ache.

"Would you like a happy ending?"

Gulp.

Watch yourselves in the mirror as your hand strokes his erection. Feel how nicely the skin of his shaft slides over his stiffness. Take your time and watch his face as you stroke him. *"Mmm, I like this."*

Here's the part where you blow his mind. Ask him to show you how he gets himself off: *"Baby, would you show me how you do it?"* Assure him that you think it's hot (*it is!*), and that you want to see what he does to make himself come.

Now, watch what he does. Let him focus on the sensation of being held by you while he masturbates. Whisper encouraging things to him: *"That looks so good . . . I love watching you do that . . . you're making me so hot."*

Now reach around and try your hand. Remember the speed he used and how tightly he gripped himself. Brace yourself for his orgasm. When he seems close, whisper, *"I want you to come for me."* When he does, catch as much as you can on your gloves. Don't forget to sneak a peek in the mirror while it's happening.

Once he's finished and his breathing's returned to normal, take off the gloves, toss them aside, and give him *the look*. He may be spent, but that doesn't mean it's over.

Because every girl—deserves her own happy ending.

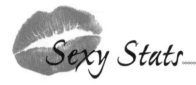 Sexy Stats

- The website www.handjobadvice.com provides free instructional videos on many hand job techniques, such as "Milking the Bull" and the "Wild Butterfly."

- The Thai fingernail dance, "Fawn Leb," is performed on special occasions, such as when greeting honored guests. Using slow and elegant hand and wrist movements will assure your guy that he's pretty special, indeed.

- Shania Twain raised a few eyebrows when she wore a pair of black, fringed opera gloves and over-the-knee boots during her "Man! I Feel Like a Woman" performance at the Grammy Awards.

- Gloves have been at the forefront of fashion since Napoleon. Some famous Americans with a thing for gloves: Jacqueline Kennedy Onassis, Marilyn Monroe, Audrey Hepburn, Madonna, Christina Aguilera, Dita Von Teese, Miss Piggy, and every Miss America, ever.

No. 6 SATIN STROKES

INGREDIENTS
1 pair of elbow-length or opera-length gloves
1 satin nightgown or slip
sexy shoes
1 full-length wardrobe mirror

YOU'RE GOING TO RUIN A PAIR OF GLOVES THIS week. And it's going to be *so* worth it.

I talked with a lot of people while researching this book, and while I wasn't surprised to find that massage is a popular romantic activity, I was amazed to find out that there are places around the world where women give massages while wearing gloves. I'm not talking about household gloves, either. Full-length, satin *opera gloves*. Wow. Now *that* is something special. *That* is something worth trying.

Gloves enhance a woman's arms, wrists, and hands—some of the most expressive parts of her body. In Thailand, there is a national dance that highlights the beauty of those parts: the fingernail dance. Young women perform this gracious and elegant dance while wearing six-inch-long brass fingernails covering the tips of their fingers. Dance is connected with the beliefs, traditions, and customs of Thailand and plays an integral part of the country's culture. You can't visit Thailand and *not* feel welcomed, especially if you watch a group of young women performing the fingernail dance.

This week you too will let your fingers do the talking. But you'll be wearing a great pair of gloves.

They don't *have* to be satin; there are sexy latex and leather gloves available as well, in different colors and lengths. Most adult boutiques have something suitable, or search online to find a pair. Midweek, leave the gloves someplace he'll notice them, like draped over a chair or by the phone in the kitchen. If he asks you what they're doing there, smile and tell him, *"They're for Saturday. For your happy ending."* And leave it at that.

Saturday, after dinner, excuse yourself and go to the bedroom. Set the mirror about three feet from the edge of the bed and dim the lights. Step into your lingerie and shoes, and then pull the gloves on. Walk out to where your sweetheart is, straight up to him, and stroke a finger under his chin in a come-hither motion. Kiss him and say, *"Follow me."*

In the bedroom, *slowly* undress him in front of the mirror. As you do, exaggerate the movements of your hands. They are encased in gorgeous gloves, and every flourish you make with your wrists and fingers is dripping with seduction. Extend your arm and drop his shirt. Hold your arm out a bit longer than necessary. Tease him as you walk around him. When his pants have dropped, lead him backward till he is sitting on the edge of the bed with his feet planted on the floor, and stand between him and the mirror.

Now run your hands across his skin, tracing his collarbone, circling his nipples, raking your fingers up his thighs and continuing to the tip of his penis. He's going to love how cool and smooth and sensual it feels, and he's going to be *hard*. Get behind him, straddling his body with your legs. *"Look at that,"* as you snake your

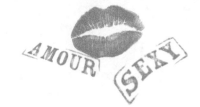
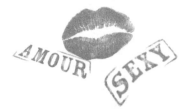
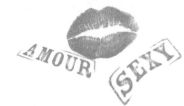
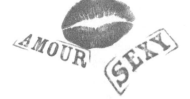

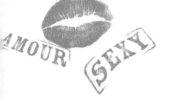
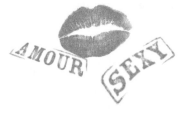
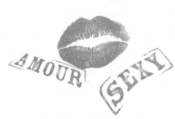

seduction no. 7

Warrior Princess

ISRAEL

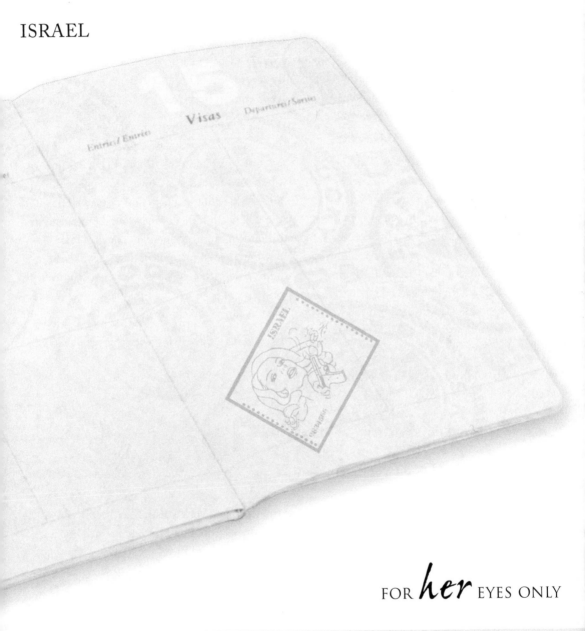

FOR *her* EYES ONLY

$

for him. Picture a pattern of color on them, then open your paint cans and make it happen.

You might feel silly at first, but get past it. Go with the music. Imagine yourself as a model for a major artist, as a gift for your lover. Circles here; stars there. A splash of blue; a stripe of gold. Nothing is permanent. You can paint over your mistakes. And you can go as far as you want, turning yourself into an explosion of skin and color.

Ready? Cover yourself with a light button-up top, a cardigan sweater, or a loose cami. Call your guy to the bedroom. *"I have a treat for you,"* you tell him with a twinkle on your eye. *"Close the door."*

Now pull off your shirt. Give him a moment to take in the amazing view. Then, before he's had time to gather his shaken thoughts, walk up to him, put your hands on his shoulders, and push him against the wall. Drop to your knees and tug his pants down, just to the top of his thighs, so that he's partially bound by them. Be aggressive. Grab his penis and tug on it. Make it hard. Take it into your mouth and work it until you hear him panting and moaning, but don't let him finish, not yet.

With your hand firmly locked around his erection, lead him to the bed. Shimmy out of your own pants and lie down on the bed. *"Get on me,"* you say. *"Put it in, now."* There's a common belief that the person on top is the one who is in control, but that is not really true, as you are about to prove. You're in a position that's so often derided as boring, "plain vanilla" sex, but today you are clearly the aggressor. Rock your hips hard, hard enough to lift him in the air. Lock your calves around his thighs and use your leg muscles to pull him deeper into you. Sink your fingers into the flesh of his butt and squeeze, pulling his cheeks apart in sync with your crazy hip thrusts.

Your guy will be overwhelmed, overjoyed, overloaded. The woman he loves has clearly put a lot of effort and thought into seducing him. She's used herself as a canvas, made herself into art. Her newfound glory is on display, right there beneath him. Her newfound erotic energy is bouncing him around like a sex toy. Her newfound strength and confidence will last, he hopes, long after she pulls a ferociously powerful orgasm out of him, which may, under these wild circumstances, take only moments.

He's going to love living with this new Warrior Princess.

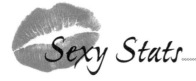

Sexy Stats

- Body painting's sexy appeal isn't new. In 1933 at the Chicago World's Fair, Max Factor and a female model were arrested for causing a public disturbance when he painted her with his new line of movie makeup.

- Female Israeli soldiers can disassemble and reassemble an M-16 assault rifle in 30 seconds. Just imagine what they can do with *other* weapons.

- *La'isha,* the Israeli magazine for cosmopolitan women, reports that 72 percent of Israeli women know where their G-spot is and are able to climax during intercourse.

- In Israel, many modern brides (and some grooms!) receive mehndi (the henna stain body art made popular by Madonna) as a symbol of blessings, joy, and beauty.

No. 7 WARRIOR PRINCESS

INGREDIENTS
body paints and brushes
hot music
cold wine (optional)
bedsheets you don't mind getting messy

AMERICAN WOMEN ARE GENERALLY PERCEIVED as strong and independent. *Cosmopolitan* magazine even has an award for Fun Fearless Females. But when it comes to real-world standing-in-the-face-of-danger *fierceness*, few cultures can rival the women of Israel.

And you can't say they didn't earn that reputation. They go on to lead normal lives, just like women everywhere, but for two wild years, when they're barely adults, they share one big common experience that has a powerful impact on them: *They're warriors*. Almost all of them have served in the military. Even the mildest, sweetest Israeli girl, the one who teaches art class or raises babies can fieldstrip a gun or dig a foxhole. She can knock you on your butt, bare-handed. More to the point, she has had to stand toe-to-toe with the guys in their army, and as any female soldier anywhere in the world can tell you, that gives you some serious self-confidence. Time spent as a warrior teaches you to stand tall. It teaches you to grab life and enjoy it while it lasts. A couple of years of that will make you into one strong, proud, kick-ass woman, no matter what you go on to do with your life.

You're going to show your man some warrior attitude this week—and he will be blown away by it. The actual seduction will be (as it is so often in military life) a *quickie*, but you're going to spend some time preparing for it. You're going to practice a modern Laura Corn version of a ritual that warriors have been engaging in for centuries. You're going to *paint yourself for battle*.

Not the famous green-and-black jungle camouflage paint of modern soldiers, or the black under-eye stripes of football players. No, I'm thinking of something just as fierce but much more feminine and much more beautiful. You're going to *paint your breasts*. You're going to tap in to your creativity. You're going to turn your body into art. And if you want some inspiration, just search online for photos from Boombamela.

Every spring, young Israelis gather at the beach for Boombamela, a festival that's part Woodstock, part Burning Man, part Passover celebration. Inevitably, breasts come out, and paint goes on, but it's remarkably unlike the drunken boobs-in-the-camera riot of your typical spring break. These women are *proud* of what they're showing. They're cool about it. And if you aren't cool, if you show too much horn dog attention, then too bad; you don't get to look anymore. (And you do *not* want to be walked to the exit by an Israeli girl's male friends.)

So prepare for a private Boombamela of your own. Pick up some skin-safe paints and a couple of brushes. A glass of wine might put you in the mood, as well as some moving music. Stand in front of your bathroom mirror, take off your top, and look at yourself. Not all women are happy with their breasts. *But your man loves yours.* He worships them. He may not say it out loud, but he considers himself incredibly lucky that he has a pair of breasts right there in the same house with him, breasts he can sleep next to, breasts he can touch. So dress them up a little

seduction no. **8**

The Naughty Chair

GREAT BRITAIN

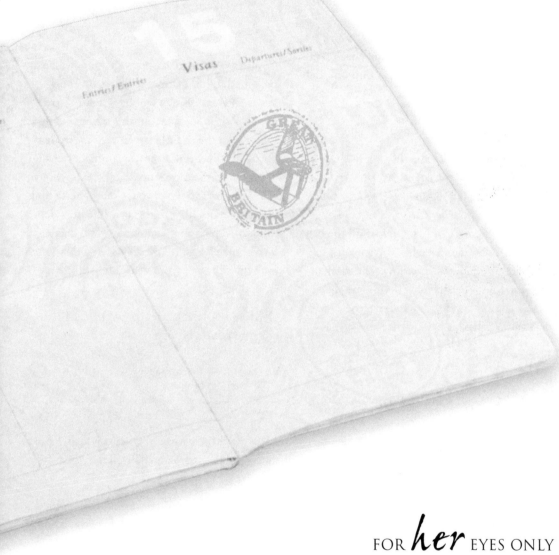

FOR *her* EYES ONLY

$$

nibble it, right through the fabric. *Oh. My. God.* What a view. The hat, the red lips, the white teeth, the lingerie. And then suddenly . . . *what's that sound?* Oh, yes, he knows that sound. It's a vibrator. You had it hidden between your legs, and now you've turned it on, buzzing it against your clit while he watches you drag your teeth across the taut fabric. After a minute or two, bring the buzzing toy to your lips and kiss it. Invite him to lean over and kiss it, too. *Yum.* Now whisper another order: *"Bend over the chair."*

Oh, *that's* naughty. Stand up and make him lean forward over the chair's padded back. Walk around behind him. Compliment him on his lovely *arse.* Run your nails across his bum and don't be afraid to dig in. He's tough back there. Give him a pinch, a spank, and a giggle.

Pull his underwear down to his thighs. *"Ooh, look what I found!"* you squeal, as you wrap your fingers around his dangling jewels. *"I bet you'd do pretty much anything I say right now."* Laugh as you give them a gentle squeeze. Pull the belt from your robe and tickle his bottom with the silky fabric. Glide it up and down the crack of his bum. Run it between his thighs and tie it loosely around his erection, tugging the ends of the sash to make his penis dance and his sack

jiggle. *"Oh! I should keep this tied here* all *the time! Whenever I think you're not listening, I'll just give it a little pull . . . like this."* Ulp.

You have his full attention. The smooth, shiny fabric, knotted around his shaft; the submissive position; your awesome, amazing outfit and strong sexual persona—no wonder the Brits love these bedroom games. It's all so sexy, and it allows your man to slip into an erotic reverie. He'll do anything you say because it just feels so bloody good and he doesn't want this fantasy to stop.

Give him two more orders, which he will be delighted to fulfill. First, tell him to get on his knees, in front of the Naughty Chair. You're going to sit in it again, but this time it won't be the back of the chair between your parted legs, but rather, his head. Enjoy his ministrations. Take your time; there's no doubt about who's in charge here. And when you're ready, make him lift your ankles high in the air while he slides inside you, pumping and rocking and making love in the chair until the two of you thoroughly soak the silky belt from your robe, still tied around his tool.

Oh dear. I hope it's machine washable. That's going to leave a bit of a mess.

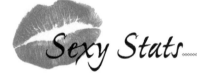

Sexy Stats

- In 1963 Lewis Morley took an infamous photograph of Christine Keeler (the Monica Lewinsky of her day, as she nearly brought down the British government with an affair). Keeler sits backward in the chair, naked. And naughty.

- More and more people are experimenting with spanking, since the sting causes the brain to produce feel-good chemicals. What's more, aficionados say there's a direct link between a slap and a man's prostate and a woman's clitoris.

- It might not surprise you to learn that the Rabbit vibrator is the most famous sex toy in the world. At Ann Summers, a popular sex toy chain in the UK, Rabbit sales are over one million a year. One of their Rabbit models, in addition to stimulating the clit and vagina, also sports an anal stimulator. Have you ever had a *Trigasm?*

No. 8 THE NAUGHTY CHAIR

INGREDIENTS

1 chair
1 red bra with matching knickers
1 red lipstick
3 sheets of paper
1 vibrator

1 slinky robe, with belt or sash
1 pretty hat
1 pair of high heels
1 soft blanket or throw

I *LOVE* THE BRITISH ATTITUDE TOWARDS SEX! Sure, their Queen still seems all proper and reserved, as she should be. (Though who really knows for sure? Maybe she's got her staff trained to stay out of the palace when they see a sock hung on her giant gold doorknob.)

But her subjects? They are wildly open about sex. They joke about it, talk about it, and buy the most fabulous outfits just to participate in it. Truly, some of the hottest kinkwear on the planet comes from England. And my jaw dropped when I read the British statistics on role playing, spanking, vibrator ownership (highest in the *world*!), and bondage games.

Fact: you can't spell f**k without the UK.

You're going to be one seriously naughty kitten this week, with this collection of British kink. Naturally, you will need *red lipstick*—luscious, wet, and shiny. Early in the week, apply it to your lips and press a perfect red lip print onto three sheets of paper. The first one gets folded over and left in your lover's car, with no words at all. That single kiss will be enough to put a smile on his face and get him thinking about you for the rest of the day. The next day, leave another paper kiss where he will find it, with this sultry note: *I've got plans for you, if you're good. Or if you're bad*. Let him find the third kiss on Friday morning: *Tonight. Bedroom at 8. No sooner, no later*. It will be a wonder if he gets any work done at all this week, with your lips on his mind.

The moment he walks into your bedroom, there is room for only one thought in his head: *You look gorgeous. Amazing. Hot*. You're straddling a chair in the middle of the room, with the back of the chair facing him. Your arms rest on the top of the chair's back, and your bare legs are spread wide. He can't really see the middle of your body, because there's a soft, luxurious blanket draped over the chair's back and seat, making it quite cushy for you but blocking his view.

What he *can* see takes his breath away. The highest of high heels. The reddest of red lips. You're wearing a hat—which, like all hats, has the magical power to transform you into another character altogether. In a voice barely loud enough to be heard, you say, *"Come here. Stand in front of me."*

Now he can see the rest of your naughty outfit. Under a slinky, open robe, you're wearing only panties and a bra. In red, of course. Be bold. Smile as you pat his zipper. Undo his belt and slowly slip it free from the loops. Timeless dominatrix move: fold the belt in half and *crack it*—and watch him jump. Open his pants and let them drop to the floor. Leave his underwear on and continue to massage his growing shaft. Now give him an erotic image that will be burned into his brain for the rest of his life.

Pull his cotton-clad erection to your mouth and kiss it. Yes, put a bright red lip print right on his briefs, directly over his twitching penis. Kiss it again, and again. Pull it into your mouth and

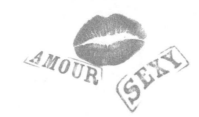

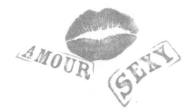

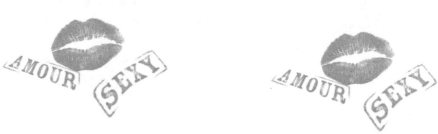
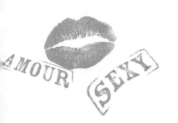
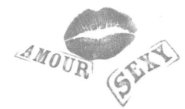
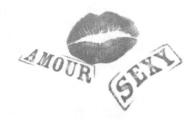
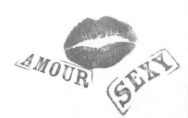

seduction no. 9

Undeniably Sexy

CUBA

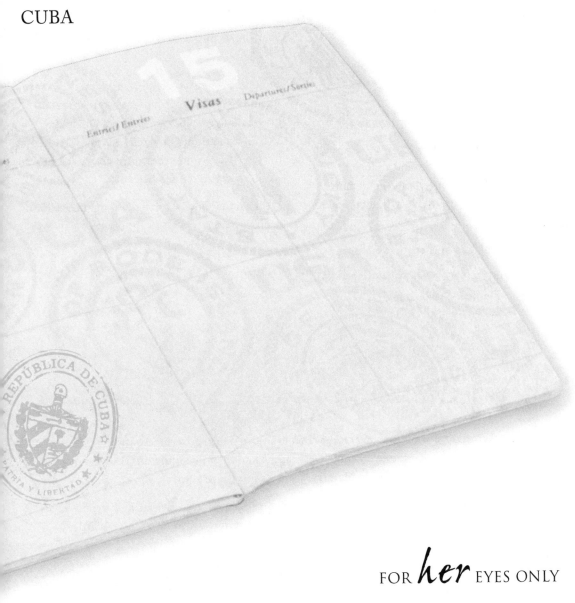

FOR *her* EYES ONLY

Tell him to undress while you watch, and then to lie on the bed. With the music still pumping, strip very slowly, taking off everything except your jewelry. Crawl up his body toward his face, your nipples grazing his skin, his erection between your bodies. Straddle his head and lower yourself to his mouth. Close enough so your lips touch but not too close. "*Kiss me here.*" Keep your clitoris just in front of his tongue. "*That's it, that's so good . . .*" Sit straight up and focus on moving only your hips until he's squirming beneath you.

Are you sweating yet? You *should* be. Your skin should be slick and dewy. Slide your body down his chest toward his *chile.* When you reach it, stay there, rubbing your wetness into his shaft. Lean forward like a jockey and slide onto him. Hold very still and tense your vaginal muscles around his penis ten times slowly, then rapidly ten times.

Watch his look of surprise when you do.

Slowly sit up and move your hips in time with the music. Don't worry about sliding up and down yet; the sensation of your tight wetness pulling him in all directions will amaze him. Raise your arms over your head as you ride him, so the bracelets fall together and jingle.

Whatever you do, don't let him finish yet. The role of *jinetera* is to keep the *bestia* under her control. When his body signals that he's close to coming, lift yourself off quickly and continue your dance on his tongue. From shaft to tongue, you control him with your hips and your PC muscles.

Remember that you are in charge and don't stop teasing him with your hips and your kitty until he's shaking with the effort of holding back. While you're riding him, tell him you want him to come. Keep your eyes locked on his and never let up your grip on his shaft.

He'll wonder how sex so wild—could leave him feeling so tame.

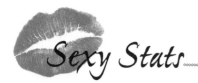

Sexy Stats

- Cuban women love sexy, revealing clothes that even the Cuban government issues military fatigue miniskirts to its state workers to wear on the job. There's nothing like being sternly questioned by a customs officer in high heels and a super-short skirt!

- Cuban women take great pride in their appearance. In fact, not to wear earrings is considered unfeminine and a signal that the woman is not interested in sex with men. There is little discretion in this.

- The nineteenth-century explorer Sir Richard Burton wrote that if a woman can master the technique of *pompoir*, or stimulating a man's penis using only her vaginal muscles, "her husband will value her above all women."

- In a poll, nearly all Cuban women described themselves as "optimistic" and "creative." Good news for Cuban men in the bedroom, *sí*?

No. 9 UNDENIABLY SEXY

INGREDIENTS
1 tight-fitting outfit
1 pair of heels
several skinny metal bracelets
large gold hoop earrings

CUBAN HIPS DON'T LIE.

In a country where the average salary is $18 a month and a pair of jeans costs $80, Cuban women make do with what they have. And what they have is one hell of a sexy attitude. Tonight, you'll be taking on the role of a Cuban seductress and riding your man like a wild beast.

If there's one thing all Cubans young and old share, it's a love of Salsa. Salsa music and dance is a huge part of Cuban culture. (You thought it was cigars? Well, cigars do have their place, but that's another seduction. Ahem.) Cuban girls know how to move their hips, thanks to Salsa. They grow up knowing exactly how to drive a man wild sexually. And that's just what you're going to do, when you ride your lover like a beast who needs taming.

Tonight, with your hips and your pelvic muscles, you will perform a dance of seduction and you will conquer your man. When you speak during the day, slip in a *"Gracias,"* a *"Sí, señor,"* or an *"Adiós"* at the end of a phone call. Just to tease.

When you dress for tonight, leave the PTA skirts in the closet. Squeeze yourself into a tiny miniskirt or short shorts, a halter top with plenty of cleavage, and high heels. The goal is to look sexy, not perfect. Do you have belly rolls? Yeah, well, most of us do. Cuban women know that every size and shape is sexy, and use their extra flesh to their advantage.

Wait, what are you saying, Corn? I'm saying *flaunt it.* Do a sexy walk in front of your mirror: shoulders back, ass out, hips *working it.* The more confident you are, the sexier you seem.

Tonight you want to sparkle for your date. Use shimmery body lotion. And since Cuban women are conscious of their sex appeal 24/7, adorn your body with jewelry. Wear gold or silver hoop earrings. Slide on a bunch of tiny metal bangles, too, the ones that jingle when they fall together.

To set the mood, put on some Cuban music and turn up the thermostat. This is a night in Havana, baby, and Havana is *muy caliente.* Mix yourselves a couple of Cuba Libres (That's Rum and Coke), set your guy in a chair, and start moving your hips to the beat. He doesn't care if you're dancing authentic Salsa Cubana or the Electric Slide at this point; you're shaking your assets for him, and that's what gets him hot.

Now, this is important. He may be the beast, but you're the jockey. You *own* him. You *control* him. You point him to where you want him to be. And where does a *jinetera* want to be? On top, of course.

Look at him over your shoulder while you dance. Let your eyes tell him what you're thinking, *I am in control. I am going to ride you. I am going to tame you.* You're feeling it now: the power of the seductress. Between kisses, whisper how badly you want to feel him inside you.

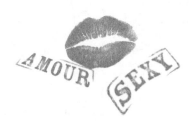
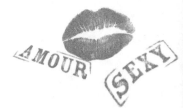
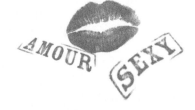

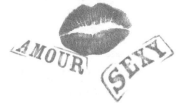

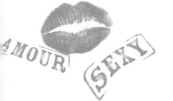
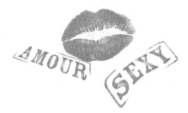
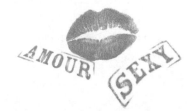
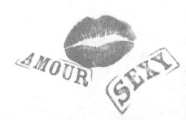

seduction no. 10

Wah-Wah Wow!

USA

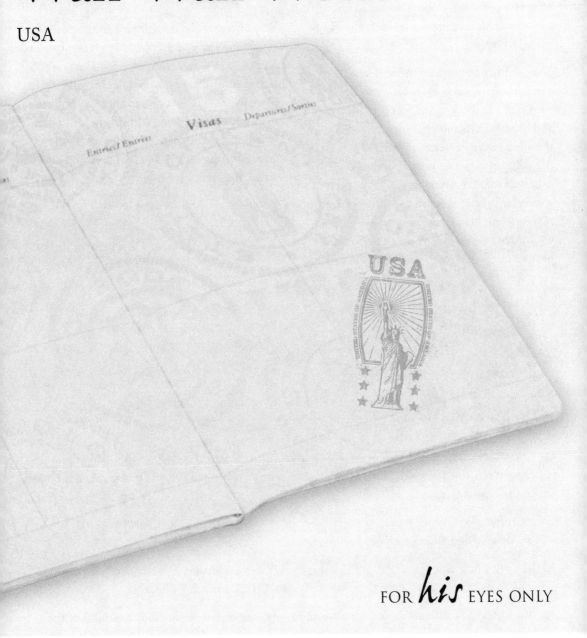

FOR *his* EYES ONLY

Hold up your gift bag again. Let her watch you reach into it and pull out the *other* toy. Oh, wow, she's thinking; this is getting interesting. Turn it on low, like the first vibe, and stroke her with it. Stroke her with the other one again. *Then stroke her with both*. Hold them parallel and glide them alongside her clitoris, just for a moment. She might gasp; the sensation is intense. Turn up the speed on both machines and use them to draw patterns on her.

You don't need to explain the science of it to her, but your smart new friend *constructive interference* is about to swagger into the room and help you make things crazier. Speed up the vibes even more, but tune them so they are not quite on the same note. Feel the beat? That wah-wah sound is even more intense when you feel it pounding your hand. The slow pulse of interference is more than noise now. It's a visceral shake—and you're about to use that power to shake up your lover. Press the two

toys against her once again, on either side of her swollen clit. Send that powerful *wah-wah-wah* beat through her. Slide the toys up and down her lips. Put one of them inside again, just two inches deep, right where her G-spot is now screaming for relief; put the other one outside, near her clitoris, and *oh . . . my . . . god* the pleasure is strong, overwhelming, bigger than anything she has felt before. The beat of the fighting vibrations picks her up and carries her, taking her to a place where she can no longer control her body, and doesn't want to. A place where she can only curl her toes and arch her back and ride along with the pulses, a place where she might say dirty things and not even remember them. A place she'll want to visit again, and take you with her.

I hope you bought rechargeables.

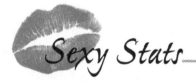

Sexy Stats

- The clitoris is the only organ whose sole purpose is to give sexual pleasure. The head of the clitoris contains approximately eight thousand sensory nerve endings, the greatest concentration in the human body.

- Victorian doctors used steam-powered vibrating devices to treat women for "Hysteria." Seriously? Paging Dr. Feelgood.

- The Hitachi Magic Wand Personal Massager, available worldwide, is one of the best-loved devices by women and couples, and is often called "The Cadillac of Vibrators."

- The U.S. states of Alabama and Mississippi ban the sale of devices intended to stimulate the genitals.

INGREDIENTS
2 vibrators with adjustable speed controls (bullet vibes work great)
1 gift bag

IF YOU'VE EVER TUNED A GUITAR, OR TAKEN A ride in a twin-engine boat, you're familiar with *beats*. That's the *wah-wah-wah* effect that happens when two sounds are close in pitch but not exactly the same. It's the sound of two notes fighting each other. Scientifically, it's called *constructive interference*.

I'm not an acoustic engineer, so I'm not that interested in complicated explanations of sine waves and amplitudes; I'd rather talk about orgasms. Or to be more precise, using science to help you create . . . The World's Most Powerful Orgasm. ("*BWAH-HAH-HAH-hah-hah-hah!*" cackled the horny mad scientist. "*Oh, no*," cried the helpless maiden, "*Not another powerful orgasm!*")

You will require *two* vibrators to create this extraordinary treat for your sweetheart. They should be one-piece units, so that they are easy to handle, like drumsticks. Critical feature: They should have an *adjustable speed controller*, not just an on-off switch. Shout-out to the inventor of the G-Spot Vibe and its knock-offs! That's the perfect design for this experiment, and cheap, too; I've seen them for less than $15. Days before your seduction, test your vibes. Make sure you can tune them to the same pitch. (And, as always, wash them thoroughly. Hey, that's just good sex-toy manners.) Put them both into a pretty gift bag, and if you want to make a real impression—and impressions *count*, don't ever forget!—use a velvet bag.

Early in the week, ask your sweetie for a date. It can be fancy or as simple as take-out dinner at home. The important thing, from a woman's point of view, is that you plan something rather than nothing. That sounds astonishingly simple, but it's the difference between romance and being taken for granted. Or, to put it another way, it can be the difference between let's go to sleep and let's screw like weasels. Here's another easy trick that can make a woman feel like taking off her sweats and putting on her nightie: *straighten up the bedroom*. Whoa, wait, don't toss this page! I'm not saying you have to change the sheets or, heaven forbid, actually clean the place. Just make the bed. Put your stuff in the closet. Light a couple of candles.

It won't be long before your girl is happy and aroused and sprawled in bed. Slip down between her thighs and work some magic with your tongue, and then, after a few minutes, reach for your gift bag, hidden under the bed. Hold it high and smile. You don't have to say a word. Just reach in and slide out *one* of your new toys. Turn it on low. *Ahhh.* What a lovely sound. Every woman adores it. Don't apply the buzzer straight to the clit; it's much too soon for that. Instead, draw a loop around her whole vulva, slowly circling in toward her lips. Alternate between your tongue and the toy, gradually ramping up the intensity of your action. Take one of her labia into your mouth while stroking the other with the vibe. Tease her. And then . . .

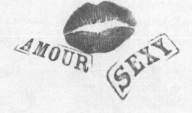

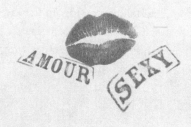

seduction no. *11*

Best. Day. Ever.

BRAZIL

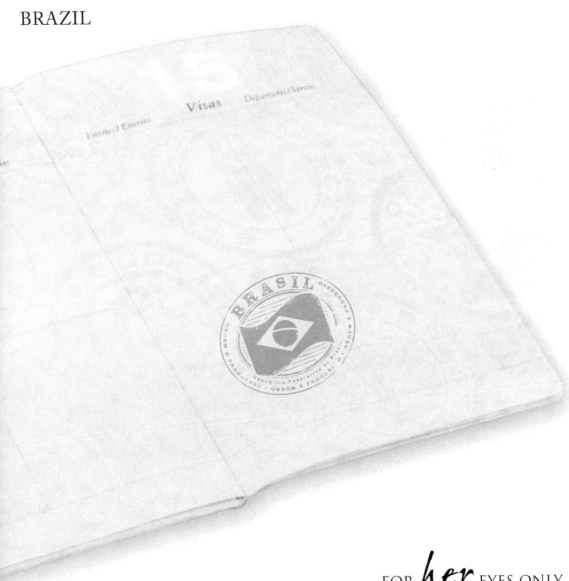

FOR *her* EYES ONLY

yourselves. You're going to find out *just how many orgasms you can have in one day.*

Believe it or not, there's more to this seduction than fun and lubricant and bragging rights. Intimacy is a two-way street: Happier couples enjoy better sex, and better sex leads to happier couples. *Oxytocin,* the hormone released when you have an orgasm, modifies the brain in a way that enhances love and trust. But you already know the results, in your heart as well as your head. When you and your mate are having great sex, problems seem smaller, compromises easier, conversation sweeter. That's a phenomenon that can last for days.

Prepare for a marathon of gratification. Tell your guy to bring home lots of snacks. Get fresh batteries for your favorite sex toys, and buy a *muito grande*—very large—bottle of personal lube. Lock the doors and turn off the phones. Remember to pace yourselves. And . . . *go.* Do it together the first time. Then do it apart. Do it

together a different way. Let him watch you do it yourself, then observe and learn as he shows you how he flies solo. Do it as often as you can, taking breaks for nourishment and laughter. And keep score of your climaxes. Not as a competition—because *you* would win that race, hands down, right?—but as a goal. Whatever number you've achieved, see if you can go one higher. At the end of the day, you will fall into an exhausted, satisfied sleep next to the happiest *cavalheiro* on Earth.

Tomorrow, go mark this date on your calendar. Hearts, stars, exclamation points, whatever. Your friends don't need to know what it stands for. (Well, maybe your very best friend.) But *you* guys will know. Every time you look at it, you'll smile and think *Feliz Dia del Orgasmo.*

Happy Orgasm Day!

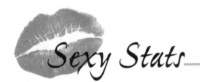 *Sexy Stats*

- *Carnaval* means "farewell to the flesh" and is notoriously wild precisely because participants are expected to forgo earthly temptations for Lent, right after the party is over. Last call!

- Like a Cher concert: A Brazilian girl may change outfits during a date just to hold your attention.

- Guys have spontaneous erections throughout the day and night, with an average of eleven during the day and nine overnight. Seems a shame to let all those go to waste.

- The Brazilian version of Valentine's Day, *Dia dos Namorados*, is celebrated on June 12. Orgasm Day is May 9.

- A world apart: according to *The Penguin Atlas of Human Sexual Behavior*, Brazilians put an average of thirty minutes into sexual intercourse, three times longer than the Thais.

- So Why Are There No Statues Of This Man? Town councilman Arimatea Dantas proposed Orgasm Day in Esperantina, Brazil.

№ *11* BEST. DAY. EVER.

INGREDIENTS
1 uninterrupted day
1 or more sex toys (optional)
personal adult lubricant (mandatory!) like Wet or Astroglide

BRAZILIANS ALREADY HAVE A REPUTATION FOR throwing the biggest, hottest party on the planet. Their notorious Carnaval—actually, dozens of huge parades and festivals—draws visitors from all over the planet. It's the last chance to indulge in the pleasures of the flesh before swearing it all off for Lent. And *meu Deus*, do they indulge! On one wild weekend every year, almost anything goes, so long as it's done *atrás do máscara*, behind the mask.

Even without the annual amnesty of Carnaval, Brazilians are known as touchers. Touching, in fact, is all a young guy might get out of his Brazilian girlfriend. On the one hand, the culture prizes virginity until marriage, and on the other hand, there's Carnaval, and the thong, and those gorgeous beaches and sexy music. The inevitable compromise is a whole lot of fully dressed not-all-the-way foreplay, and the *meninas bonitas* of Brazil are masters of it.

Reminds me of high school.

But even with the parties, the hot outfits, the dancing and affection and bare booty *everywhere*, you don't necessarily get satisfaction. You could make a pretty good argument that all the famous Brazilian eroticism is really just a big tease. (Yet again, another reminder of high school!) That might be what the city fathers of Esperantina were thinking when they established an astonishing new official holiday:

Orgasm Day.

No parades for this festival, I'm afraid. (But can you imagine what one would look like?!) Orgasm Day is devoted to raising levels of awareness about the importance of orgasms and, more specifically, to the problem that women aren't having enough of them. For all the famous machismo and seductive powers of Latin men, too many Brazilian women just aren't getting the thrill they need, and so once a year the village of Esperantina hosts discussions, lectures, and a performance of *The Vagina Monologues*. I was surprised to learn that the Portuguese word for vagina is . . . *vagina*.

Could it all be a ploy by the Esperantina Chamber of Commerce to bring in *turistas* and their dollars? Are the promoters simply hoping that they could personally enjoy a bumper crop of climaxes? Why, *sim*, yes, of course! But that doesn't make it any less of a fabulous idea. I think the honorable mayor of Esperantina is a genius. And so I say: Happy Orgasm Day! That's the message you're going to deliver to your sweetie this week, in preparation for an event that will be one of the great memories of your lives.

Orgasm Day will be something you giggle about years from now, a memory that will still put a grin on your guy's face when he is ancient and wrinkled. Tell him to clear his calendar for Saturday (and also to, um, *stop practicing* and start saving his energy). You two are going to go for a personal record. You're going to outdo

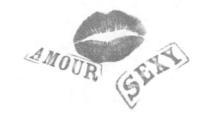
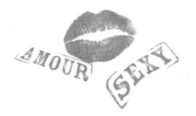
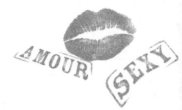
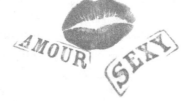
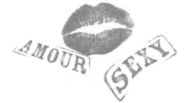
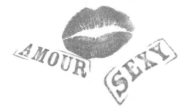
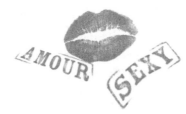
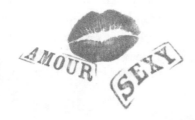
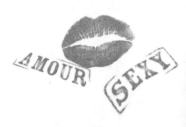

seduction no. **12**

Sweet Control

ISRAEL

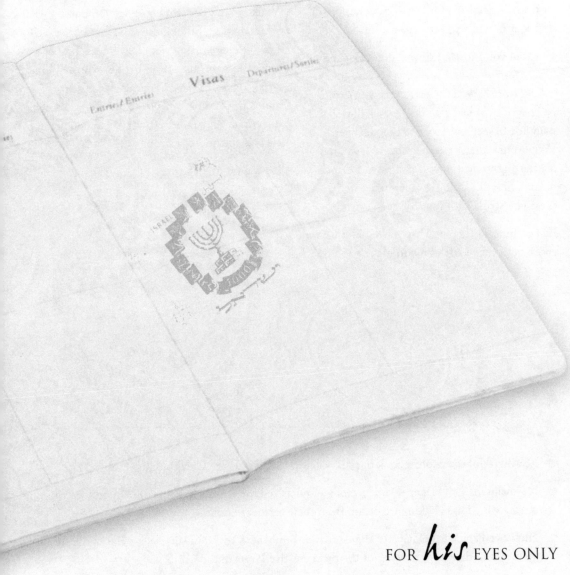

FOR *his* EYES ONLY

close to her so she can feel your heat, and with your fingers lightly trace the skin of her neck, shoulders, and nipples through the fabric of her robe. Untie the front and let it drop to the floor. *Shivers* . . .

Watch her face. Listen to her breathing. Then move the frozen bar close to her body. Trace the very same path you did with your fingers, but this time drag the tip of the treat along her skin instead. Be prepared for her to gasp, jump, flinch, and squirm while you take your time.

Use your voice to send shivers down her spine: "*Your skin is so soft . . . your nipples get so hard when I touch them . . . you look so sexy with your eyes closed* . . . Wield the curved stick like a paintbrush; see how easy it is to maneuver? Write your name across her body. Maybe things are starting to melt now, leaving sweet drips behind. She thinks you're going to erase the chocolate swirls with your tongue. *Don't.*

By this time she knows what you're holding, and you're both excited. It's time to make good on your promise of dessert. Stand in front of her and touch the tip of the treat to her lips and pull back. Tease her with the ice cream. "*Show me your tongue.*" Then let her have a lick. Keep the treat in front of her mouth, just out of her reach. Watch her mouth as she searches for it, letting her have a lick. Pull it away and take a few bites yourself. "*So good. I bet you'd like a bite, wouldn't you?*"

Walk around her as if you're contemplating what you'll do next. Stop directly in front of her. Tell her, "*Open your eyes.*" Give her the last bite of ice cream, kiss the taste from her lips, and say, "*Take off my clothes.*" You've been direct, confident, and commanding. You've made her feel excited, uncertain, vulnerable, and very sexy. Enjoy the view as she undresses you.

It's sex-on-a-stick time.

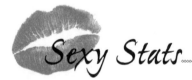

Sexy Stats

- Marilyn Monroe wrote a book of poetry called "My Sex Is Ice Cream." How tasty is *that*?

- Ice cream maker Häagen-Dazs has long emphasized the sensual delights of its products with ads showing lovers licking ice cream from their partner's bodies.

- The Love Parade is held every August in Tel Aviv, where Yotvata Dairy sells some of the freshest ice cream in the world to some of the most creative lovers in the world.

No. *12* SWEET CONTROL

INGREDIENTS
ice cream bars or other frozen treats on a stick
1 small plate
1 big attitude

TONIGHT'S SEDUCTION IS ALL ABOUT ORDER and control. As much as women want to share responsibilities with you, there's a little part of us that really likes it when you take charge. For this seduction, you're going to channel the sexual energy and power of the Israeli man.

You're already a sweet and loving guy, secure in your masculinity and your bedroom skills, but today you'll be taking it up a notch and tapping in to the raw sexual energy of the Mediterranean. Israeli men are *sexy*. Maybe it's the hot climate, or the compulsory army service, but when their passion and confidence combine—*boom!*

Early in the day, plant the seed of tonight's seduction with your partner. Tell her you've got a surprise for her and that you want her to play along. When she agrees, look her straight in the eye and in your most commanding voice say, "*I'll be taking care of dessert tonight.*" You don't need to give any more information than that. For now, let her think you're being a typical, predictable guy and planning to let her have *you* for dessert. She'll think she's got you all figured out.

Call or e-mail her later with more details: *Dessert will be served in the bedroom at 8:30. You should be standing in the middle of the floor, naked under your robe, with your eyes closed.* Be direct. Be confident. She'll be completely turned on by the thought of waiting for you, even if she doesn't know why she's there.

Pick up a box of ice cream bars on your way home. I think Dove Bars are perfect: yummy chocolate (which you know is the closest thing to sex for many of us), smooth vanilla ice cream, and a rounded, easy-to-grip stick.

You'll appreciate the shape of the stick later; trust me. Stash them in the freezer when you get home.

Look at her pointedly during dinner; keep your cool, even if the anticipation is killing you. It's definitely killing *her* knowing that you're up to something. Go about your evening together as usual, but catch her eye from time to time and wink. She likes that you have a secret.

When dessert time is getting near, walk behind her and whisper, "*Don't forget, dessert reservations at 8:30!*" Be smooth and confident. Once she's gone, get your supplies ready. Place napkins and ice cream bars on a plate or tray. Everything in order. Stand tall, shoulders back. You are in control of the situation. You are cool and your hottie is waiting for you.

Walk confidently into the bedroom. Tell her to keep her eyes closed and ask if she's ready for her dessert. Stay in character! She might giggle or ask what you're doing. She's naked underneath her robe, blinded, and nervous about what might happen next. Good! She's nervous with anticipation, and that's *exactly* what you want.

With her eyes closed, unwrap the ice cream bar. Make a lot of noise with the wrapper. Stand very

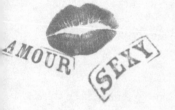
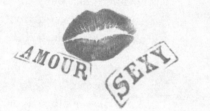
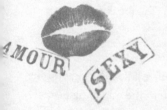
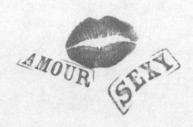

seduction no. **13**

Torn

BELGIUM

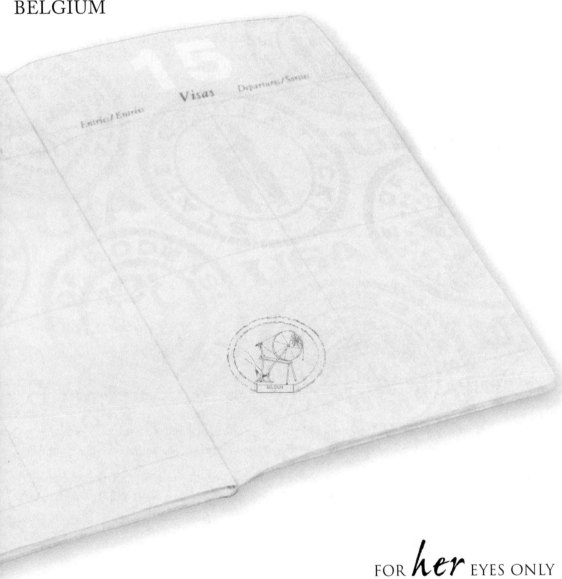

FOR *her* EYES ONLY

Push him onto his back and climb up his chest. Kneel over his face. *"I was worried about wearing them in public,"* you say, *"because you can see right through them. Can't you?"* Kneel closer to his face. Bring your lower lips within inches of his own. *"Can you see my pussy right through them?"*

Push your nylon-covered mound against his mouth, and moan. Back off, catch your breath, then push again, harder. *"Oh, that feels so good. I think you should keep that up."*

Rock your hips. Bounce a little and let him hear the pleasure in your voice. By now, he will have noticed a flaw. There's a small hole, a rip, right on the center seam. He doesn't need to know that *you* put it there, hours ago, before you even pulled the stockings on. But his tongue has found it and made it obvious.

Reach down between your thighs and slip the tips of your fingernails into the hole. Tug the edges farther apart, then press your unwrapped flesh even harder against his mouth. Let him

hear you gasp. *"I want you in me!"* you tell him, and soon he will be, his hard shaft ripping the seam apart, the tight fabric scratching and squeezing his erection on every thrust. Your warmth and wetness are more than a gift unwrapped. For him, they're a treasure taken, a secret exposed. Tonight, you've given him so much more than sex. Your actions have validated his most secret hope: You find him so irresistible that you can't wait for intimacy. You think he is so sexy that you would rather rip your clothes than put off sex for one more second. For a man, there is no higher compliment than spontaneous sex.

Even if you had to plan it yourself.

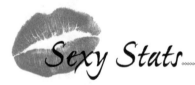

Sexy Stats

- Are stockings a male fetish? According to Freud, they are. He viewed women's hosiery as the ideal article for male fetishism since he considered a woman's legs as a pathway to her genitals.

- Here's a sampling of magazine titles devoted to hose and lingerie fetishes: *Black Garter, Black Lace, Black Satin, Black Silk Stockings, Lingerie Libertines, Nifty Nylons, Nylon Jungle, Silky Sirens, Slip and Garter, Stocking Parade,* and *Velvet Touch.*

- According to *Marie Claire,* the people happiest with their sex lives live in Belgium.

- Belgium's Cette brand is relatively new in the world of hosiery (1988), but the original company was founded in 1958 in the small village of Flanders, twenty miles west of Brussels in a historic textile area.

No. *13* TORN

INGREDIENTS

1 pair of sheer-to-waist pantyhose, in any pattern or texture
1 pair of scissors
1 thigh-length sweater
1 pair of heels

BELGIANS LOVE SENSUAL FABRICS. THEY HAVE a history with fabric that goes back hundreds of years; it was a giant industry for them, back in the days of the great sailing fleets. And even now they have an appreciation for luxe on a loom. They love silk, they love lace, they love . . . *pantyhose.*

Yes, pantyhose. American women have been moving away from them for fifteen years, but Europeans in general, and Belgians in particular, wear them often and enjoy showing them off. There are blogs (and yes, quite a few fetish sites) devoted to the beauty and sheer sexiness of women wearing hosiery, in every color and pattern, whole and shredded. I was especially moved by the work of famed Belgian photographer Rik Scott, and after I saw how outrageously gorgeous his models looked wearing pantyhose, the thought hit me:

I've never used pantyhose for sex. Not in my personal life, or in any of the five-hundred-plus seductions I've written. I've always been a stockings-and-garter-belt girl. I posted the pantyhose question on my iVillage.com page, and—Holy Hosiery, Batman!—the answer was a resounding yes. American men *love* the look of pantyhose! American women seem to think of them as merely practical, but American men agree: *Pantyhose are hot.*

The men I talked to told me about prom dates and secretaries, schoolteachers and MILFs, and sneaking glances up long, long legs made shiny and smooth by tight nylon. My friend Marty describes pantyhose as *giftwrap* over the sexiest present in the world. What a great image! *C'est si sexy, non?*

So . . . are you ready to sacrifice a good pair of pantyhose for a great lay?

Get your guy to agree to a date this weekend. On the night of the date, early in the evening, start walking around the house in an outfit that you will probably think is unfinished, and he will think is totally arousing. On top, you're wearing a long sweater, one that ends right at the top of your thighs. On bottom, you're wearing nothing but pantyhose. Sheer-to-the-waist panty hose, a bit more expensive but, according to my sources, the sexiest thing on the planet. Your girly bits are mostly hidden under the sweater, but as you walk around the house, your man will quickly start to notice that you are practically naked under there. Practically, but not *quite* naked. And that is one of the sexy secrets to pantyhose.

Flirt with him. Make sure your sweater hikes up. Have him sit on the sofa while you pose for him and dance for him. He'll be hypnotized by the sight of your bottom, your labia, your bush, all pressed together behind the barely visible fabric. Sit on his lap and ask if he likes your new hose. Kiss him while he tells you how much he loves the way they fit. Ask if he wants a better look.

seduction no. **14**

Blue Magic

BERLIN, GERMANY

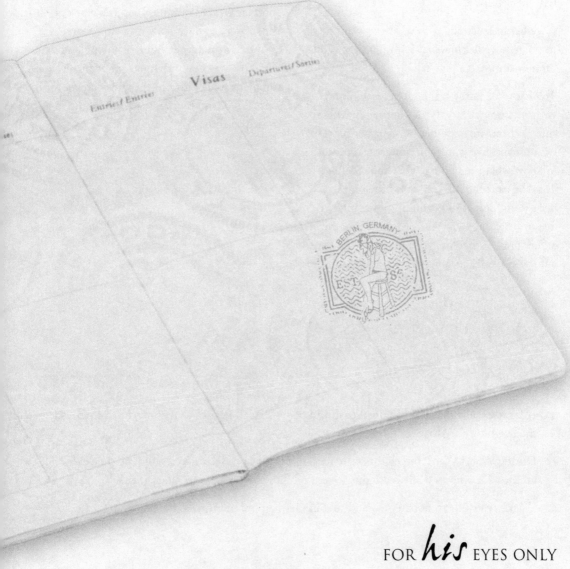

FOR *his* EYES ONLY

$

see *her*. Go outside to a private area where you can see her through the window, but make sure she's facing away from you. Then call and tell her you're watching her, you *know* every move she makes, every sigh, every naughty gesture. Tell her you're right outside the window, but she can't turn around. Instead, you want her to remove her clothes, slowly . . . *very slowly* . . . yes, that's right. You want to see more, *more*, you want her to play with herself . . .

Give her instructions as to what you want her to do: remove her bra, play with her nipples, take off her panties. It's *your* call.

Tell her to open the box of goodies and play with whatever sex toy tickles her fancy. Make sure to stimulate her emotions, stir her passion with provocative words and phrases. You want to know what she's doing, what she's feeling. That she can't see you is a total turn-on for her—doing something naughty, knowing her man is watching her. Ask her to massage the oil on her breasts, then between her legs. Tell her to put the silk scarf around her eyes and continue touching herself. Sneak out of your hiding place and let her know you're standing in front of her. Then, before she can say anything, grab her hand and let her feel how hard you are. No matter what language you say it in, *It's showtime!*

Remove the scarf from her eyes and ask her to kiss your penis, then run her tongue around the edge before drawing you into her mouth, sucking and lapping until you can't stand another X-rated minute. Then trade places with her so you can have sex with your cabaret girl on the chair with her riding you long and hard. You'll be so sexually charged you won't need *any* stimulant (blue pills or otherwise) except for the sensual blue light wrapping you both up in an erotic paradise.

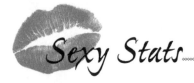 *Sexy Stats*

- A female masturbation machine boasting a penis-shaped pedal was manufactured in Dresden at the height of the Roaring Twenties.

- During World War I, blue lights were used in France and Belgium to signify higher-class brothels for officers while red lights were used for lower-ranking military men.

- Viagra-type pills were patented and sold in German pharmacies in the 1920s.

No. *14* BLUE MAGIC

INGREDIENTS

2 cell phones with hands-free sets
1 or 2 blue lightbulbs
vibrator, dildo, and/or other sex toys

chair
silk scarf
goody box

*W*ILLKOMMEN, *BIENVENUE*, WELCOME TO THE cabaret!

Remember that old film with Liza Minnelli? Blue light, smoky club, angst-filled music in the background. And right in the middle of the stage sat gorgeous Liza in her peekaboo black stockings and snappy garters, her long legs astride the chair like she was riding her favorite stud to paradise.

You could *smell* the sex in the air.

Set in Germany during the Weimar Republic, it was that wild, raucous time between the world wars when the Teutonic male indulged in every sexual depravity he could stick his penis into: live sex shows, his and hers masturbation machines, make-out cubbyholes in seedy dives, spanking paddles, and a nightclub decked out with two hundred telephones at numbered tables. Here you could engage in dirty talk anonymously with the cute blonde across the room without her knowing who you were or where you were sitting.

Sooo delicious and something you *definitely* want to include in your lovemaking arsenal. This week, you're going to visit divinely decadent Berlin and indulge in an erotic cabaret that will not only have you rising to the occasion, but will give your favorite *Fräulein* a thrill with a modern twist that will put those Weimar playboys to shame.

I bet you took a peek at the ingredients, so you know it has something to do with cell phones. And, oh yes, sex toys, a silk scarf, and a chair. When the big day arrives, tell her to wait for your call on her cell phone. Then, after you've set up the seduction, call and give her directions to the spot where you've placed the chair bathed in a mystic blue light.

Put the chair in an empty spot with enough room around it to set up the blue lightbulbs. Use standing lamps set at an angle—*indirect* lighting is more flattering. When she sits down on the chair, the blue light effect on her psyche is immediate. Erotic, sexy urges will sweep over her as its sensual effect induces a mood of playfulness, sensuality, and blissful arousal. She'll feel like a Hollywood movie star basking in the blue light, known by directors to spark a lively mood during a love scene.

What could be more dramatic and enticing?

Make sure the goody box is within her reach. You've filled it with the sex toys and other fun, sexy items like a feather, massage oil, incense sticks, and aromatic candles. Still on the phone, tell her to sit in the chair and wait for your call again. *But,* you tell her, she's not to open the box until you give her the okay. Then hang up. She won't be able to take her eyes off the phone, just waiting for your call.

Pick your peep show spot beforehand. Make sure it's somewhere she can't see you but *you* can

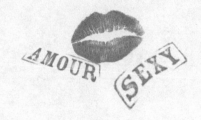
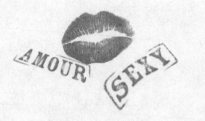
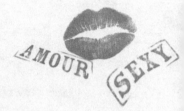
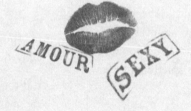
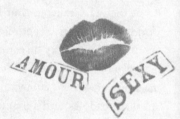
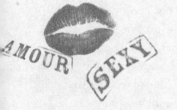
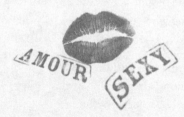
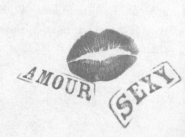

seduction no. **15**

Girls Will Be Girls

THAILAND

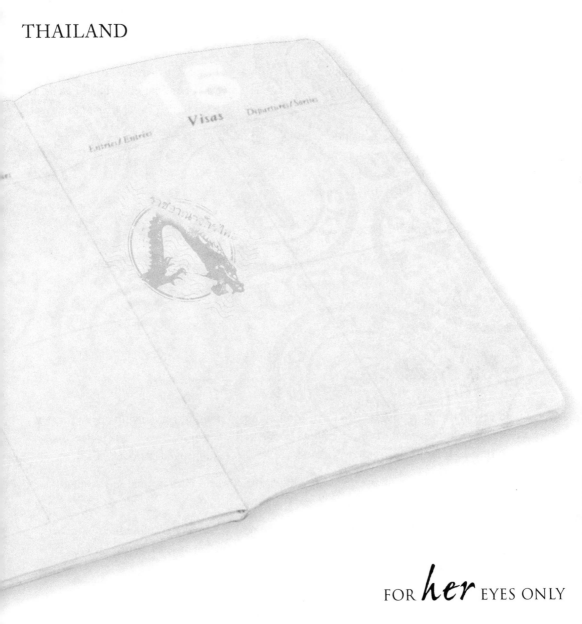

FOR *her* EYES ONLY

some cushions, and lie down on the floor. And he'll do it; oh, yes he will, because he *knows*.

Now that he's flat on his back, take a little stroll around him. Toss your skirt around; let him get another peek. Place your foot on his chest and give him a good long look up your legs. Step over his head, facing toward his feet. Dance to the music. Watch his eyes moving back and forth, following your hips and cheeks as they rock to the beat. His favorite thing in the world, the most precious part of his favorite person, is *right there*, floating before his eyes. And now it's getting closer.

Ooh, yes, much closer. Your knees bend and your slow swaying dance brings your hips and your bottom down close to his face. His upskirt fantasy has become much wilder now; he's not just looking anymore, he's *right up there*, under your dress, feeling your thighs brush against his

cheeks. He is wrapped up in a universe with boundaries defined by your skirt, and a center that is nothing but your own sexual pleasure.

But he's not there alone. Go ahead, get comfortable. Drop to your knees while keeping his grinning face right between your swaying thighs. Lean forward, grab his belt, and give him a hand. And then some lips. Don't undress him, just unzip him. Take him into your mouth and start trading kiss for kiss, lick for lick, orgasm for orgasm. His upskirt fantasy just became *your* fantasy, now that he's exploring the wet, delicious treat you've been hiding (well, *almost* hiding) all evening long.

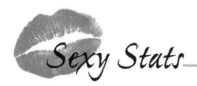 *Sexy Stats*

- The most famous upskirt shot is of Marilyn Monroe. Who could forget the white dress that she wore when she stood over the subway grate in *The Seven Year Itch*? It lasted only a few seconds, but that shot sealed her fame forever. Today, skirts are short and paparazzi are *skilled*.

- The upskirt peek is popular all over Asia and the Pacific Rim. So much so that mirror-toed shoes have been spotted in the streets. Tsk-tsk!

- Can can dancers at the Moulin Rouge wore white crotchless pantaloons under their petticoats, causing gentlemen in top hats to lose their heads when the mademoiselles leaped into the air and landed in a split.

- Another (less innocent) peek underneath a gorgeous blonde's skirt: Sharon Stone's police interview scene in *Basic Instinct*. Now there's a woman who knew something about the art of distraction.

INGREDIENTS

killer shoes (remember, he's going to be spending most of this seduction focused on your lower half)

2 smooth legs

1 neatly trimmed puss

1 flouncy, flirty skirt

0 panties

TATTOOS, NIP SLIPS, AND BAD BOY DATES aren't enough to get you into the Hollywood spotlight anymore. The bar has been raised. These days, a celeb who wants to generate an explosion of camera flashes has got to get caught in public without her panties. It's become so common that there's even a name for it: the *upskirt shot*. Actresses used to boost their careers with a *Playboy* spread; now they spread their knees for YouTube supremacy.

And it works. It works because a peek up your dress can make a man headspinning crazy. Naked is one thing. But a glimpse of actual bare snatch on an otherwise fully dressed woman? That's a gift from the locker-room gods. It's like he's getting away with something. As upskirt royalty Paris Hilton used to say, *that's hot.*

But Paris (and Britney and LiLo and the rest) didn't invent it. The act—no, the *art*—of publicly flashing your privates was perfected some years ago in the wild no-taboo nightclubs of Bangkok.

The bar girls of Thailand are known throughout the world for an intriguing blend of old-world propriety and anything-goes immodesty. To Western eyes, they appear both respectful and daring, sweetly demure yet giddily uninhibited. There's no better place to see this heady mix in action than in the notorious Soi Cowboy area, and at its heart—assuming you can even get into this white-hot spot—you'll find a happy crowd in the Dollhouse A gogo. Young women in pretty party dresses dance with one another on a balcony over a nightclub floor. *And the balcony is transparent.* You can see through it. Delighted couples sit below, looking right up through the clear floor, watching the underwear-free dancers overhead. Cameras have recorded the spread of the upskirt phenomenon from Bangkok to the rest of the world.

And this week it's coming to your home.

You're going to be showing off your kitty, and so you've got to get her groomed. Trim, shave, or wax her into shape, and then look for the perfect outfit for her unveiling. You want a skirt that moves and flows like a beautiful theater curtain. As with most good seductions, this one starts with a Coming Attraction to get your audience in the mood. It's a simple preview: Sometime early in the evening, maybe even before kids and company have been shooed away, take your guy to a private spot, grab his hand, and pull it under your skirt, all the way up. *"Hey, guess what I forgot to put on today?"* you whisper, and then . . . walk away.

You've officially short-circuited his brain. Now he *knows*. Whatever else might be going on—dinner, phone calls, cleanup—he's thinking about that sweet little secret hiding under your dress. He wants to see more. But like the happy, laughing, exquisitely beautiful Thai girls who inspired this seduction, you are in control. And when you're ready to begin the show, you can tell him to put on some music, dim the lights, grab

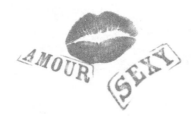
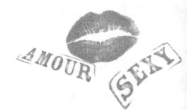
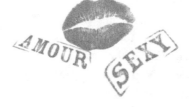

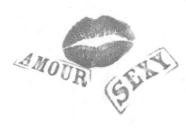
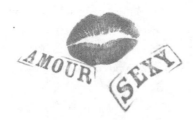
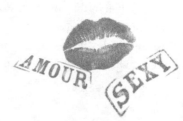

seduction no. 16

French Kiss

FRANCE

FOR *his* EYES ONLY

$$

chocolate candy, I mean. Yum. Delicious. Also a remarkably effective method of foreplay.

Saturday, launch a fusillade of kisses her way. (And if the opportunity presents itself, throw in a kiss-related Bum Bite! Bite her bare ass before she gets dressed. It's a guaranteed laugh, and it will leave her thinking about your mouth all day long, every time she sits down.) Tell her to meet you in the living room at sunset for some more kissing surprises.

And here's the gorgeous sight waiting for her when she meets you at home. The setting sun fills the room with a fiery glow. The light sparkles through a bottle of champagne (of course—*bien sûr!*) and the two thin glasses next to it. Freshly rinsed strawberries glisten like fat rubies on a plate. You've tossed a blanket on the floor and piled pillows against the sofa to make a comfortable backrest. It's such an easy scene to set, but for her, it's the very essence of romance, the climactic scene of all the best chick flicks rolled into one. Tell her to go get comfortable and then join you for some Strawberry Kisses.

When she comes back, snuggle next to her and make a big presentation out of popping the cork. The bubbles dance in the late afternoon sunlight as you raise your glass and make a toast to her beauty. Hold a strawberry up to her lips; let her take a bite, and then . . . *try to steal it back with a kiss.* Sip, nibble, kiss again. Repeat those three steps until clothes begin to disappear.

The French were really on to something when they created champagne. The fizz makes magic, and the subtle *brut* dryness is a perfect balance for the sweet, plump strawberries. The combination inevitably leads to what Americans call French Kissing. Wet, flirty, deep kisses let you share the flavor—and share your excitement. And they don't have to be limited to your girl's mouth. Apply a dab of fruit to her nipple and kiss it. Pour a splash of champagne in her bellybutton and lap it up. Keep moving in that direction and soon you'll be enjoying what the French call Australian Kissing.

That's a French kiss . . . *down under.*

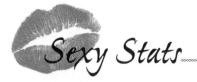 *Sexy Stats*

- Champagne Oral Sex: The bubbles stimulate nerve endings, increasing skin sensitivity. Cheers!

- During passionate kissing, what does a man pass to a woman that puts her more in the mood for love? Answer: testosterone. That's why we get so turned on.

- But now it's a feature: Bubbles were once considered a major problem in champagne production, causing bottles to explode while aging. The wire collar that secures the cork was invented by a monk named Dom Pérignon.

- A pair of Czechs hold the world record for continuous kissing—42.5 hours.

- France has 20 different words for kissing.

- Sitting in a Tree: July 6 is International Kissing Day.

- And it means the same thing over there: The French word for the number 69 is *soixante-neuf.*

No. *16* FRENCH KISS

INGREDIENTS
1 bottle of champagne
2 pints of strawberries
1 blanket
pillows

W**HAT DO WOMEN REALLY WANT?**

Men have been asking that question since the dawn of time. Back then, the answers were obvious—*a little fire, a little shelter, and would you be a dear and slay the saber-toothed tiger that's been stalking the tribe? Thanks so much, honey.*

But ever since things settled down and we got civilization and plumbing, men have often found themselves mystified by women's desires. I can tell you what women want, though. I've interviewed more than two thousand women for my books, and talked to hundreds more on radio and television. All over the world, women say that what they want is . . . *more kissing.* In surveys, kissing often shows up as the number one turn-on for women, and women everywhere believe they don't get enough of it. With one notable exception.

France.

The French apparently get *all* the kissing they want. La République Française is, in fact, the Oral Nation. Her citizens take great pride in the various ways they have made high art out of anything that makes use of *la bouche*, the mouth. Dinner can last for hours. *Talking* about dinner can last for hours. And if you ever get a sommelier on a rant about the glories of French wine, the sipping and slurping and tasting and smelling, well, you're not going anywhere for a while. With all that focus on oral pleasure, it's no surprise that kissing is high on the agenda for *les amoureux* of France.

And this week, kissing—in all its wonderful forms—is going to be the focus of your entire seduction.

Start with some Surprise Kisses—delivered out of the blue, for no special reason, accompanied by a smile and a squeeze. You score a lot of points with a Surprise Kiss, and yet it requires no preparation at all. (Other than brushing your teeth, plus mints or mouthwash, but you knew that already, didn't you? Of course you did. I'm just saying.) The Surprise Kiss is so touching because it demonstrates that you're thinking of your sweetie *even when you don't want sex.* Women find that . . . startling. And thrilling. Thursday, give her a Necklace Kiss. Start on the neck, just below her ear, and plant a circle of light pecks down her collarbone and around her neck, finishing up with a nibble on the other ear, a.k.a. the Earring Kiss. Don't follow up with a move toward sex, though. Let her enjoy the anticipation that comes with slow foreplay.

Sometime during the week, go for the We Interrupt This Call Kiss. When she's on the phone with a friend, grab the handset and say, *"Could you hold for just a moment?"* Plant a big, passionate kiss on your girl, tell the caller, *"Thank you!"* and hand the phone back. Yes, they will be talking about *you* for a while. All good.

Friday, add an Ice Cube Kiss to the mix. Just like it sounds, the Ice Cube Kiss means surprising her with your frosty lips. After dinner, be sure to give her a Hershey's Kiss. The actual

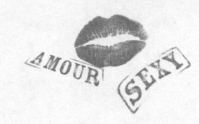
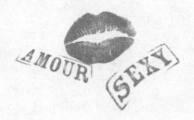
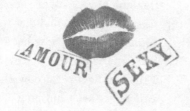

seduction no. 17

Hello, Lover!

NEW YORK, NEW YORK, USA

FOR *her* EYES ONLY

$$

When your baby walks into the room, smile innocently and say that famous Carrie line, *"Hello, lover!"* He's looking at you, stunned. He's never seen shoes like those, except in the movies. Wiggle your toes and run your fingers across the feathers. He totally wants to. Lean back and drop both knees to one side, keeping your shoes on the mattress in front of you. *"What should we have for breakfast?"* Offer him just a peek at your panties and then slowly move your knees to the other side. Bring your knees together, look up at him, and spread them apart slowly, exposing your barely covered pubis and keeping your fancy slippers together.

He may be so flabbergasted he doesn't speak. That's all right, Ms. Innocence, you can ask for what you want. Ask him to take off your panties and hand them to you. Bring them to your nose and inhale. It doesn't matter that you've had them on for only a few minutes. He loves your scent, and *watching you do this will turn him on.*

Extend a leg, dangling the slipper from your toes. *"Do you like my shoes?"* Offer your leg to his caresses, bringing the tickly feathers into contact with his skin. *"Aren't they soft?"* Help him undress but leave your camisole and shoes on. Keep that visual contradiction, even during foreplay. Run the feathers up the inside of his leg while standing, go down on one knee and take him into your mouth, keeping a shoe out where he can see.

When you're both ready, climb onto his erection and ride him slowly. *Keep your shoes on.* They've transformed you into a hot, sexy, innocent vixen. He's going to have a lot of trouble staying calm when he sees them in the closet tomorrow.

Good news: These shoes, like episodes of *Sex and the City*, are just as fabulous the second or the third (or fourth) time around.

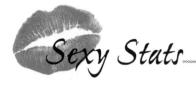

Sexy Stats

- Saks Fifth Avenue's shoe department in Manhattan has its own zip code: 10022-SHOE.

- Men love sexy shoes. Sure, "do me" pumps are a popular choice, but the strappy sandal wins hands down with men. The reason? Toe cleavage: the cracks between your pretty toes at the front of a pretty sandal. Now, that's cleavage we can all flaunt!

- According to an *Allure* magazine study, the average American woman owns 27 pairs of shoes.

- A recent British study suggests that men get aroused simply at the sight of women's shoes. So leaving your sexy pumps in the middle of the kitchen might not be such a dangerous thing, after all.

No. *17* HELLO, LOVER!

INGREDIENTS
1 cotton camisole
1 pair of sheer panties
1 pair of marabou slippers (preferably pink or white)

QUICK, WHAT'S THE FIRST THING YOU THINK of when you hear the name Carrie Bradshaw? Okay, *after* sex.

That's right, *shoes*. Thanks to Carrie and *Sex and the City*, women around the world know who Manolo Blahnik and Jimmy Choo are. We may not be able to afford their designs, but we know them. From strappy sandals to pointy-toed sling backs, shoes that cost hundreds of dollars aren't something you can overlook in a story line. And whether you are a Carrie Bradshaw fan or not, there's no denying the sex appeal of shoes.

There's an episode in Season 6 called "Great Sexpectations," where Carrie and her boyfriend Berger have hit a dry patch in their sex life. They connect passionately in public, but in the bedroom, nothing's even warm, much less hot and bothered. Carrie takes matters into her own hands by buying new lingerie and a pair of marabou slippers that will, according to Samantha, make Berger "come in his pants."

All right, Samantha Jones and her graphic imagery aside . . . *marabou slippers*? Not f**k-me pumps? Not thigh-high boots? Nope, Carrie gets the most frivolous, fluffy, fabulously *feminine* footwear a girl can own. To spice up her sex life. Why? For goodness' sake, my Barbie doll had marabou slippers, and we all know she and Ken *never* did it.

Why should New York City's most famous sexpert need another pair of shoes to create romance? Because Carrie is, as all of us are, a set of contradictions. She's sophisticated and she's goofy. She's intelligent and she's naïve. She's independent and she's needy. She's very sexy. And she's very sweet. Carrie, despite her impossibly endless closet, isn't really different from you or me. It's all about the contradictions—naughty and nice—and for this seduction, the contradictions begin with a pair of shoes.

Get yourself a pair of marabou slippers. Try them on. Notice how quickly your thoughts of, "Who could possibly wear these shoes?" turns into "I *love* these shoes." See how pretty they make your feet look and how glamorous and sensuous you feel wearing them. Next, slide on a pair of very sheer panties, ones that show *everything*. Suddenly, you're a contradiction. Your shoes are so innocent next to those racy panties, and don't *you* feel sexy. Tuck everything into a drawer together with a demure camisole.

And wait.

Then, on a weekend morning, when he's out getting the paper or walking the dog and you have time to yourself, put on your contradictions. First the cami (sweet), and then the panties (naughty). Step into the shoes last. They're so girly, and yet they practically scream "sex." There'll be no question as to what's on your mind. Seat yourself in the middle of the bed; pull your knees to your chest and wait.

seduction no. **18**

Wrap It Up

USA

FOR *her* EYES ONLY

$

Smile and tell him to open box #1. Tell him he can wrap that pretty plastic anywhere on your body he wishes. Show him how you've bound your ankles. Cross your wrists in front of your body and suggest that he could wrap them together. But before he starts, he should know what's in box #2.

He'll be surprised when he pulls out the scissors. Let him know that once he's wrapped you up, he can cut a hole in the plastic anywhere he likes. The rule is, *he has to use his mouth on the hole.*

Oh yes, the good part is coming. And if things go right, so will you.

There's something delicious about the way your man is completely focused on you as he wraps the plastic wherever his imagination takes him— and wherever you let him. How adventurous are you feeling? Being bound is not the important part—that's just for fun. You can leave your hands free to explore other options, especially if you decide to let him take his clothes off.

The plastic wrap is soft against your skin, silky. And especially titillating on certain body parts. Tell him to lower the straps on your nightie and slide it down. Now he can wrap your breasts, and

things can get really exciting! And if you let him go lower, well, let me tell you it's a whole new sensation—WOW.

Now it's time to take out the scissors. The tips are rounded, but he should pinch some plastic between his fingers just to be safe. He cuts a small slit, maybe between your wrapped breasts . . . Oh yes, a small snip of the scissors, then his mouth there, and you're really heating up.

Do you want him to use the vibrator on you? Yes, you want it all, and he's eager to please. Because one of the hottest things for a man is seeing the pleasure he brings you.

It's time for box #3.

Have him run the vibrator over your skin. Tease yourself—and him—by not letting him get to your erogenous zones for a while. You decide where you want to be touched and if you're going to use the lube. Open your thighs a little wider and *tell* him. And when you can't take it anymore, let him cut you out of the chair, bend you over the kitchen table, and, well, *you know.*

Wrapping up leftovers will never be the same.

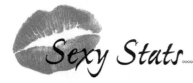 *Sexy Stats*

- According to the Kinsey Institute, those who are most likely to try bondage are between the ages of thirty and forty-four, are educated, have full-time jobs, and earn more than $50,000 a year. Bondage is smart, successful, and youthful.

- Plastic wrap was invented by accident in 1933 by Ralph Wiley, a Dow Chemical worker, but wasn't used for food packaging until 1956. I'm sure Mr. Wiley never thought of using it this way.

- Most North Americans have sex at 10:34 P.M. Doing it at eight means you're shaking things up.

- Over the last fifteen years, the number of men and women who have reported trying bondage has doubled!

No. 18 WRAP IT UP

INGREDIENTS

1 box of colored plastic wrap
1 kitchen chair
1 vibrator
your sexiest baby doll nightie

1 pair of children's safety scissors
3 gift-wrapped boxes with easily removable tops
1 tube of lube (optional)
several candles

WHO KNEW THE SUPERMARKET COULD BE sexy?

I was shopping the other day when I came across a display of colored plastic wrap: purple, pink, yellow, and blue. I was reminded of a seduction I wrote back in 2002 where my female readers wrapped themselves in Saran Wrap and challenged their men to find the elusive end. Needless to say, the guys loved it. I immediately started thinking about new ways to have fun with this stuff!

Interestingly, every year Americans use enough plastic wrap to shrink-wrap the entire state of Texas. Women are buying a *lot* of plastic wrap. And a few of us are taking it home and having all sorts of adventures.

Did you know that women are also more likely than men to introduce the idea of bedroom bondage? Don't worry, I'm not talking about leather and chains. I'm talking about *power*. And there's nothing hotter than handing that control over to your man. It will make him feel powerful. Manly. *Erect*. And when you're tied up, the only thing left to do is to lie back and enjoy. You're not responsible for anything, other than a little direction: *A few inches to the left, honey. Yes, right there . . .*

Here's how you do it.

E-mail him at work: *Come into the kitchen tonight at exactly eight o'clock. I'll have a surprise for you.*

Give yourself plenty of time to set the stage for your seduction. Place a chair within arm's reach of the counter, where you'll set the three boxes, which you've labeled #1, #2, and #3. The scissors go into box #2, and the vibrator goes into box #3, along with the lube, in case things get serious. (Let's hope they do!) Leave the plastic wrap out because you're going to use it before it goes into box #1. There are several colors available: Maybe blue goes with your eyes, or purple matches your lingerie?

Now it's time to take a long bath; rub some scented lotion into your skin. Enjoy the ritual of preparing yourself. By the time you slip into your lingerie, you're ready for the evening.

Turn down the lights in the kitchen and light some candles. Let's face it, we all look better by candlelight. At ten minutes to eight, sit in the chair and wrap a length of the plastic wrap around each ankle, binding your legs to the chair legs. You're a little wild, a little wanton, and it feels *wonderful*!

Reach over and slip the plastic wrap into box #1. You're ready. A little excited, maybe? Good.

At eight o'clock your man walks in. Enjoy the look on his face: pleasure, *lust*. It may take him a few moments to notice you're bound to the chair, your thighs parted. He knows he's in for a wild evening, and I'll bet he has a hard-on already.

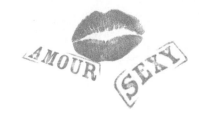
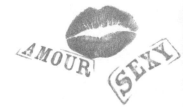
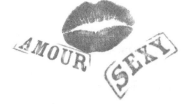

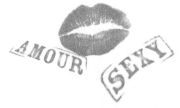

seduction no. 19

Hidden Holiday

EASTERN EUROPE

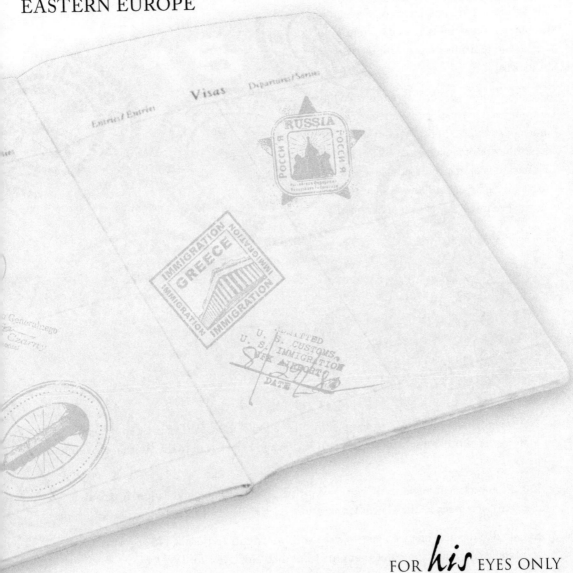

FOR *his* EYES ONLY

Her card is on the tray table. Its message is short and incredibly powerful: *Thank you for everything you do. You are my soul mate. I love you.*

Yeah, definitely tears.

Join her on the bed and hand her a gift. She'll pull off the ribbon and wrapping and smile when she sees a beautiful, elegant picture frame. The photograph inside is just the two of you. No kids, no pets, no friends, just two people in love. A moment of happiness, frozen in time. Your sweetie will remember this morning every time she looks at it.

Your job is not done. For International Women's Day, you need to shoulder some more of the burden of running a house. Make the bed, do a couple of loads of laundry, that sort of thing. But your reward is on the way. Because whenever you make a big, unexpected show of affection like this, you eventually, always, open her heart.

And, ahem, her legs.

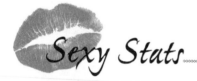 *Sexy Stats*

- Not tonight, *tovarich*, I have to get up early for the Revolution: IWD started in the United States as a political cause but caught on in Russia and helped lead to the Russian Revolution of 1917.

- But the government *wants* us to, honey: Worried about declining population, Russia has declared September 12 the Day of Conception. Back to bed and spreadski, my little Зайчик!

- But, uh, I'm the only one who gets to sleep with you, right? In Bosnia, Herzegovina, Croatia, and Hungary, women sometimes get gifts from their employers for IWD, too.

No. 19 HIDDEN HOLIDAY

INGREDIENTS
2 thank-you cards
1 flower
1 small photo frame and a picture of the two of you
gift certificate to spa, along with her card (optional)

Boo-yah! Fist bumps and high fives all around! Men of the Western world, rejoice—for you finally have an opportunity to take an official, genuine, lady-type holiday and *score points* instead of sweating bullets.

Most girlfriend holidays are sources of anxiety for guys. We women know this and want you to understand that we think it's cute how you strain yourselves trying to figure out the right gift for Valentine's Day, or our birthday, or the anniversary of the day you first said the words *I love you.* (You do remember that date, right? Right?? Oh, come *on,* it was the day I did that thing, you know, that thing you like so much . . . yeah, *that* day. Remember it, or you're never getting that thing again.)

Okay, here's the sad truth about the lady holidays. *You have to celebrate them,* but you don't get all that much credit for them. It's just part of your job. You're expected to commemorate her birthday, Valentine's Day, and the rest. Woe betide the dude who forgets.

This week's seduction holds an incredible opportunity for you. You get to honor your lover on a legitimate holiday that she most likely doesn't even know about. It's a day set aside to honor all women, but if she grew up speaking English, there's a good chance she has never even heard of it. It's International Women's Day, and it falls on March 8th. It's *huge* in parts of the world—Eastern Europe, and the former Soviet countries especially—but it hasn't quite caught on in North America yet. And that's why this is going to make such a big splash with your sweetheart. You're going to make a tribute to her . . . *and she won't even see it coming.*

Your first step is easy. Buy two nice cards, one for her, and one for her mother. *And not the same card.* We talk, you know. On her mom's card, write a sweet, simple note: *Thank you for raising such an amazing woman. I am blessed to have her in my life.* (No mom? Your girl almost certainly has a relative she adores, someone who helped make her into the woman she is; send a card to *that* person.) Mail it so it arrives just before March 8th.

You have a few other steps to take to get everything ready by the morning of International Women's Day. And you'll have to get up extra early on the eighth, because you're going to prepare the ultimate treat, the thing none of us ever get enough of: *breakfast in bed.* Coffee, juice, toast. A single flower on the tray. (In Russia, it would be a *yellow mimosa.* So pretty!) Explain that it's Women's Day all over the globe, and you're celebrating because you got lucky and found the greatest woman on Earth. Say it just like that: "*You're the greatest woman on Earth and I wanted to take a day to let you know how much I appreciate you.*"

You might see tears at this moment.

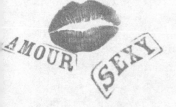
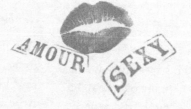

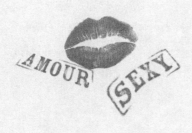

seduction no. 20

Xtra Toppings

CANADA

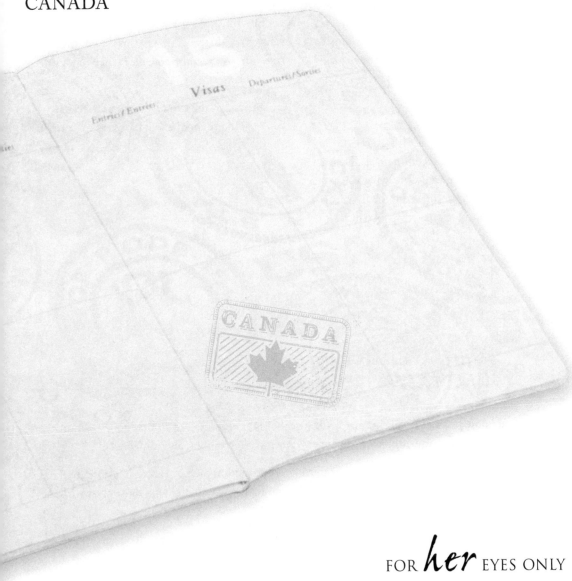

FOR *her* EYES ONLY

previews, search fields, and customer ratings. You can narrow your hunt to films recommended for couples and read what other couples had to say about them. (You can also narrow your search to an unbelievable range of fetishes and specialties. OMG.)

So promise your guy a Saturday night of pure fun at home. When it arrives, greet him in your Guy Land shirt-and-panties look. Smile. Hand him a beer and the remote. Snuggle up and let him run the TV tonight, whatever he wants to watch, while you snack on his favorite pizza. (Surprising Guy Fact: Men are wired to respond dramatically and emotionally to the smell of cheese.)

Kiss him between bites. Lick his sauced-up fingers. Make out during commercials. Distract him with occasional glimpses of what you're hiding under that big shirt. And finally, surprise him with the ultimate guy treat, dirty movies

for two. Drape one leg over his while you watch. Get into the action on-screen. Let him *see* you getting into it, nipples popping, fingers sliding between your thighs. He's in a Guy Land fantasy now, watching the woman he loves getting totally turned on right in front of him.

You know where to go from here, and if you don't, just imitate what you're watching. Become a porn star for an audience of one. Get him hot, get him off, and get ready to go again because, well, that's the way love goes in Guy Land. It's fast, furious . . . and frequent. Hence the bottle of lubricant.

Be sure to get the extra large pizza. Because you're going to *love* having leftovers tomorrow.

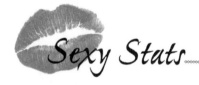 Sexy Stats

- Did you know pizza is an aphrodisiac? Not just the sight and smell of all that gooey, yummy cheese, but the basil, mushrooms, red peppers, green chilies, onions, and tomatoes.

- The French can lay claim to "the earliest pornographic motion picture," according to Patrick Robertson's *Film Facts*. The story line centered around a "weary soldier who has a tryst with an inn servant girl."

- If home videos are your thing, then head to the USA. Americans and Canadians lead the way for favoring sex in front of the camera.

No. 20 XTRA TOPPINGS

INGREDIENTS

1 pizza
6 bottles of beer (optional)
1 bottle of lube
2 hot adult movies (see sugardvd.com or videobox.com)

THEY REALLY TRY, DON'T THEY? GUYS, I MEAN. They try to understand women and give us what we want. I'm not saying they always *succeed*, of course! And they are frequently hilarious in their attempts, don't you think? But, bless their hearts, at least they are trying a lot more than they used to. It's sweet. And comical.

But for this seduction, you're going to let him off the hook. This weekend, give your guy a break from all things feminine. Set up a night of romance *manstyle*. You're taking a trip to Guy Land, a place where the seat is always up, and you can scratch whenever and wherever you need. Just don't pull any fingers while you're there.

To create this little slice of heaven on Earth, you need to get the things a guy loves most. One of those things is *you*, naturally, but it might surprise you to know what outfit he wants to see you in. Not silk or satin. Not a camisole or teddy. Sadly, you won't even get to buy a new outfit, because what you need is already hanging in the closet. *His* closet. It's a man's dress shirt. A traditional white oxford button-down, if he owns one, a shirt big enough to hang on you like a tent. Guys love this look! I've heard it in a thousand interviews. Men love to see a girl in an oversized shirt, somewhat unbuttoned, with nothing underneath but regular panties. It's one of the few things in life that is both hot and easy. In Guy Land, it counts as lingerie.

Your evening will probably require alcohol in some form. And it must not be in bright unnatural colors, come loaded with fruit, or have a name that ends in "tini" unless it is an actual James Bond shaken-not-stirred martini. Beer is fine. Beer in a glass bottle is better. Let him twist the top off for you, because, *"Ooh, you're so strong!"*

Oh, and then there's that one extra ingredient that's always guaranteed to put a smile on a guy's face. *Porn.* Adult films. I cracked up the first time I heard about that Canadian company that actually delivers pizza and porn to your home. I mean, it sounds like an Internet prank, right? Too funny to be true, I thought, but if you live in Winnipeg, you can get a dirty DVD with your pepperoni, and as I write this, the founder is looking into franchising. (I think it goes without saying that the founder is a guy, eh?) Now, I personally see one big problem with this arrangement and it's this: *you gotta look that deliveryman in the eye at your door.* Yikes! He knows! And while that's fine if you live in a fraternity house, most women I know prefer their erotica to be delivered discreetly, and that is one area where the Internet truly shines. It works just like regular movie rentals. Not only can you shop online for DVDs delivered unmarked in the mail, but you can get the movies sent straight to your computer. Straight to your bed, if you have a laptop. Best of all, the Net brings to adult films all the cool features it brought to other kinds of online shopping:

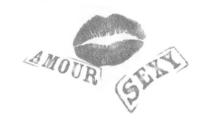

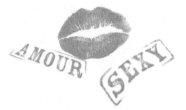

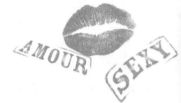

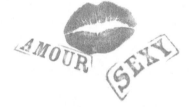

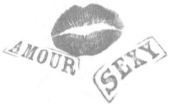

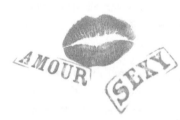

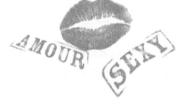

seduction no. 21

A Lesson from the Master

HOLMBY HILLS, CALIFORNIA, USA

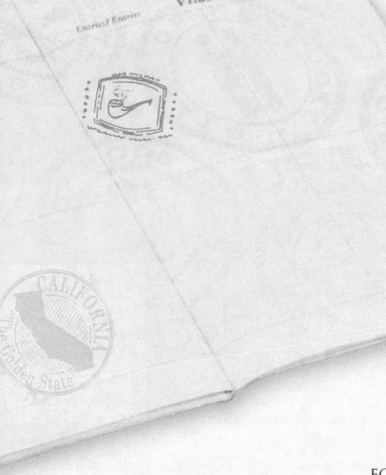

FOR *his* EYES ONLY

$$$

While your girl is putting on her shimmery new pajama top, set up your home theater. Cue up one of her movie picks. Toss some big cushions on the floor and sofa. Set out a couple of drinks. And become a Playboy for the evening. The Hefner kind of Playboy, I mean: sweet, attentive, flattering. Make your lady feel like a star. Look at her as if she were actually glowing. *"The best line is not really a line,"* says Hef. *"The best line is listening."* The Man knows what he's talking about.

Snuggle up and start the movie. Don't hit on her while the show is playing. *The silk will do the work for you.* Every woman adores the feel of cool, shiny silk. It caresses her breasts and glides across her shoulders like the hands of a masseuse. The hem grazes her bare thighs, while her long, bare legs brush up against the silk covering your own legs. The silk makes her feel sexy, before you ever lay a hand on her.

When the show is over, move in for a kiss. Slip your hands under the fabric. Let her feel your desire for her. But don't take off your pajamas.

When the time is right, let her play with you through the open fly on your PJ bottoms. Your hard-on looks even more amazing when it emerges from a field of silk, as if it were some incredible work of art or a gift on display in a fancy store. And even after she's hot and wet and ready to open her legs, keep your PJ's on— let the silk fabric surround your shaft and slide up against her thighs and cheeks when you enter her. The sensation is awesome. She knows what it feels like to wear lingerie while she makes love, but this is different. This is like feeling her partner wearing lingerie, with silk sliding up and down against her kitty, and getting wetter with every stroke; silk bouncing off her bottom; powerful masculine muscles wrapped in silk and then wrapped around her legs.

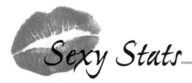

Sexy Stats

- "Pajamas are a playboy's best friend," said Hef, in his fascinating *Little Black Book*. What he meant is that the PJs and the parties and the Movie Nights and all the rest aren't just marketing tools. They are foreplay.

- What does Hef like in a film? Apparently, it's smart dialogue, adventure, unrequited love, and romance; *Casablanca* is his all-time favorite movie. The 50th anniversary of the film started off Hef's weekly tradition of classic movie watching.

- The Playboy Mansion is notorious for its parties, often happening around the pool and its famous Grotto. The mansion is also host to Hugh Hefner's Sunday movie nights, featuring something from Hef's collection of over 4,000 films.

No. 21 A LESSON FROM THE MASTER

INGREDIENTS
1 pair of silk pajamas
1 DVD

IT STARTED, AS SO MANY REVOLUTIONS DO, with one brave man.

He was a guy who had a vision. A guy who started with virtually nothing and built an empire. One horny dude who made the world a better place for *all* horny dudes. His very name conjures the sound of rock bands, squealing girls, splashing water, and popping champagne corks. I give you The Man, The Legend:

Mister Hugh Hefner.

The founder of *Playboy* knew how to throw a *par-TAY!* I was lucky enough to be one of his guests once, at the famous Playboy Mansion West. Yes, it was pretty much everything you ever imagined, one of the few truly jaw-dropping experiences of my life. Even in his twilight years, an invitation from Hef is still one of the most coveted items in the world. But the secret to his successful gatherings is not the bunnies, or the mansion, or the notorious grotto, or the ultracool guest list. It's Hefner himself.

He listens to his guests. He's attentive to his dates. He plans an entertaining evening and then goes out of his way to make sure everyone is happy. In short: *Hugh Hefner is a really, really great host.* And if he's that good at making a whole room full of people feel special, you can only imagine how good he is one-on-one.

One of Hef's long-standing traditions is Movie Night at the Playboy Mansion. You're going to re-create some of that magic for your sweetie this week. And nothing says Special Night Ahead like an actual handwritten invitation inside a pretty greeting card: *Please join me in the living room for a movie on Sunday night, after dinner. Attire will be provided.*

You're going to provide a movie . . . *and an outfit?* Wow. Okay, you got her attention with that one. Deliver the card early in the week, to give her plenty of time to think about what you have in store for her. By midweek, send her a text or e-mail asking what movies she might want to see. Expect love, foreign accents, and not a single explosion.

Sunday evening, after you've helped your girl clear the dishes, bring out a hidden shopping bag and hand it to her. Inside she will find a pair of elegant silk pajamas. Yes, silk PJs: the official uniform of seduction. They're Hef's trademark, of course; he claims to own twenty pairs of them, and they have been helping him get laid for almost eighty years, so there must be some power in them. Pick a lush, rich color. And pick them in a size that will fit *you*. That's because your sweetie gets only the top of the pajamas . . . and you get to wear the bottoms, for the rest of the evening. (If the room is cool, you can wear a robe over your pajama pants, but remember Laura's Rule of Thermostatic Attraction: *A woman is much likelier to get undressed if the temperature's on the high side.*)

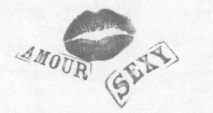

seduction no. 22

Unexpected Pleasures

NETHERLANDS

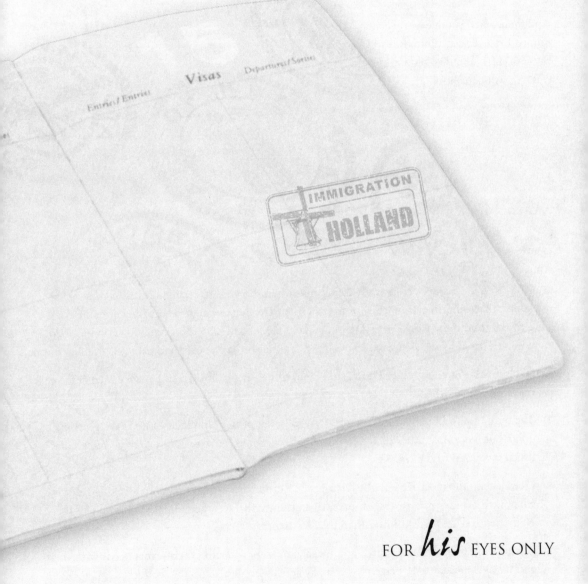

FOR *his* EYES ONLY

threads and colors are all connected, weaving the whole into a complex, rich image. You're doing the same with your woman. Weave a pattern of touches and caresses into a vibrant work of erotic art. Warm her with your breath. Strum her skin. Bring her whole body, piece by piece, into a state of happy, shimmering arousal. Stroke *all* of her, like the young Dutch masters who know so much about pleasing their young Dutch mistresses.

And then, when you have every inch of her primed for a climax, climb on. And hang on. Because she is about to blow you right out of your big wooden shoes.

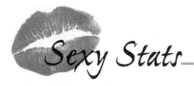

Sexy Stats

- Euro RSCG's Love & Lust study found that when it comes to setting limits for what is appropriate on prime-time television, the Dutch are, in general, far more liberal than most citizens around the world. They are more likely, for instance, to approve of depictions of hard-core sex, passionate kissing and lovemaking, and masturbation on TV during the evening hours.

- "Cold feet" is not a myth: A Dutch study found that men and women had an easier time reaching climax when their feet were warm.

- The term "going Dutch" arose in the early 1900s, out of the Dutch custom of young people going out in groups rather than one-on-one dates. Once you're seriously dating, though, it's usually the man who pays.

- Does having the most Red-Light Districts in Europe mean the Dutch are breaking records when it comes to sex partners? Apparently not, since the average number of partners in the Netherlands is 20 percent lower than the U.S. figure.

- A whopping 64 percent of Dutch adults feel confident asserting their sexual needs with their partner, as opposed to 41 percent of sexually active people around the world.

No. 22 UNEXPECTED PLEASURES

INGREDIENTS

1 date

You have everything you need. You just have to remember to use it.

WHO WOULD HAVE GUESSED? IT TURNS OUT that the most sexually liberated people in the world are the Dutch. Quiet, unassuming, immaculate little Holland has sex everywhere. In almost every statistically measurable way, the Dutch are more open about sex than any other people. Which leads to an interesting question. If nothing is forbidden, and you're getting all the sex you want, how do you keep from getting bored? How do you arouse a partner who swims in a sea of arousal?

By paying attention to the 98 percent of the body that *isn't* an erogenous zone, that's how. Dutch men know all about it. Like them, you're going to take your girl on an erotic pleasure trip this week, with lovely little detours and long scenic routes. It's a trip with a huge payoff in the end. And it couldn't be simpler. All that's required to begin your journey is a touch.

You touch your lover often, don't you? In a nonsexual way, I mean. You squeeze her hand, or caress her shoulder, or kiss her cheek at times when you are *not* specifically trying to seduce her, right? However much you do that in your normal routine, step it up this week. Hug her. Kiss her cheek before you walk out the door. Pat her on the bottom; nuzzle her neck; touch her forearm—but *do not* try to turn these sweet touches into sex. Do it, say, 20 percent more than usual, starting tomorrow morning. Seems like almost nothing, I know, but these little acts of intimacy can have an astonishing impact on a

woman. That's because we're built to respond to contact. It works like a long form of foreplay, and as you keep it up through the week, your sweetie is going to get warm and warmer.

By midweek, invite her on a date for the upcoming weekend, even if it's nothing more than a movie and popcorn. On the date, touch her often. Later that evening, when you're home and naked and finally getting hot, work a little Dutch magic on her. Here's how.

Avoid the usual patterns men fall into: back rub, which leads to sex; foot rub, which leads to sex; kissing, which leads to cunnilingus, which leads to sex. (Not that there's anything wrong with that!) In fact, stay away from tits and ass altogether, at first. Stay away from predictability. Start by caressing her shoulder . . . then move to her calf. Kiss her on the back of her knees . . . then drag your fingernails along her forearm and massage her hand. Rub the kinks out of her neck . . . then nibble the curve of her waist, just above her hips. Plant a line of kisses along her ribs and up to the edge of her breast, but skip the nipple. Glide your fingers up her thigh, but stop short of actually touching her sweet little kitty—which by now is beginning to ache for your touch.

Think of her body as one of those magnificent, priceless tapestries from the medieval Netherlands. One vibrant thread pops up *here*, and then over *there*; a certain color is visible in one spot, then another. Yet behind the art, the

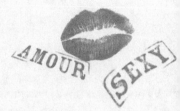
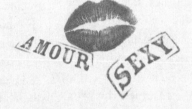

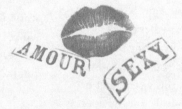
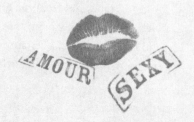
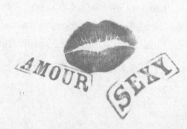

seduction no. 23

Pearl Dance

JAPAN

$

hand down to keep him hard while you dance seductively around his body.

Turn your back to him and press your buttocks into his erection, sandwiching it between your bodies. "*This feels so good.*" Straddle his leg and grind your clit into his thigh muscle. "*Mmm.*" He'll love to see (and hear, and feel) how hot this is getting you. The sensation of your slippery skin on his is heavenly, and the addition of the pearls sliding between your bodies is so sensual—a new sensation that will blow his mind.

Take off the pearls and hold them in your hand. Add soap while he watches, kneel down and use both your hands to give him a *pearl job.* Stroke his erection sensually with half the pearls in one hand, and massage his perineum and testicles with the other half. *He will not believe how amazing this feels.*

When he is close to coming, step him back into the water to rinse.

Then take his penis into your mouth and give him your full service.

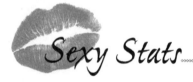 *Sexy Stats*

- Japan has been called a "sexual supermarket" and, according to 2006 statistics from the NPA (National Police Agency), the country boasts more than 17,500 pleasure playgrounds, consisting of striptease revues, peep shows, hostess clubs, karaoke bars, *and* soaplands. NPA estimates there are 1,200 bubbly palaces in Japan, offering the most expensive sexual favors of all the sex facilities.

- The Japanese tradition of mixed bathing goes back more than a thousand years, along with purification rites performed in an ice-cold mountain stream or standing nude under a crashing waterfall.

- Nude bathing in Japan doesn't receive the same attention as it does in the United States. As J. R. Brinkley, historian and editor of *Japan Mail,* once said, "The nude in Japan is to be seen but not to be looked at."

No. 23 PEARL DANCE

INGREDIENTS
creamy liquid body wash
long strand of pearls
3 bath towels

I HAVE A SLIPPERY, SEXY SURPRISE FOR YOU.

And your man is going to *love* it. You're going to treat him to a surprise visit in the shower, and you'll be using two of Japan's most famous, sensual resources: pearls and soapland.

Each year, millions of men from around the world visit Japanese soaplands to experience the most decadent erotic service in the country. This week, you are going to treat your man to the ancient Japanese art of the soapland bubble dance: Young "bubble ladies" wash men using their own bodies as washcloths. That's right, naked guy, naked lady rubbing bubbles all over him with her body. Sexy, eh? Japanese soaplands began during the era of the samurai. Not surprisingly, they became very popular places. And they are even more popular today.

I loved the idea of a soapland seduction so much that I wondered what other Japanese elements I could include for an original Laura Corn soapland seduction. Then it hit me like a grain of sand: *pearls*. Japan is the world's leader in cultured pearl production, and this week, you're going to create a surprise private soapland for your man using pearls, your naked body, and some luxurious body wash. Try one with extra moisturizers like Caress Shimmering Body Wash. Set it in the shower, locate your long pearl beads, and you're ready for this week's seduction.

One day this weekend when he gets into the shower, get undressed and put on your pearls.

Grab a rolled-up towel and join him in the shower: towel, pearls, and all.

Rak ki'i na hito ne! (Surprise!)

He is going to flip when he sees you, completely nude and wearing just those beads. But you've got a job to do, so smile sweetly and drop the towel at his feet. Turn the shower spray to the side and drop to your knees.

Oh, he's got a good idea where this is going.

Get him hard with your mouth. Don't spend too much time there; just make sure that he knows you intend to *keep* him hard. The steam rising around your bodies will open his pores and make his skin sensitive to your touch. That's a very good thing, because it's time for your pearly bubble dance.

The bubble dance is slow and erotic, and this is what has kept soaplands in business for thousands of years. Stand in front of him and squeeze the pearly soap straight from the bottle onto your chest. Look into his eyes while you spread it with your hands, lathering your breasts, belly, thighs—everywhere. Then step up with your slippery self and slide across his chest.

Use your entire body to spread the bubbles on his skin: your forearms, breasts, tummy, butt, and mound. The pearls rolling around between your bodies are so sexy and add a little massage to the mix. Focus on his pleasure, dropping a

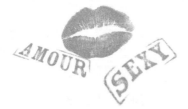

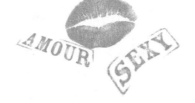

seduction no. 24

Heart Strings

FRANCE

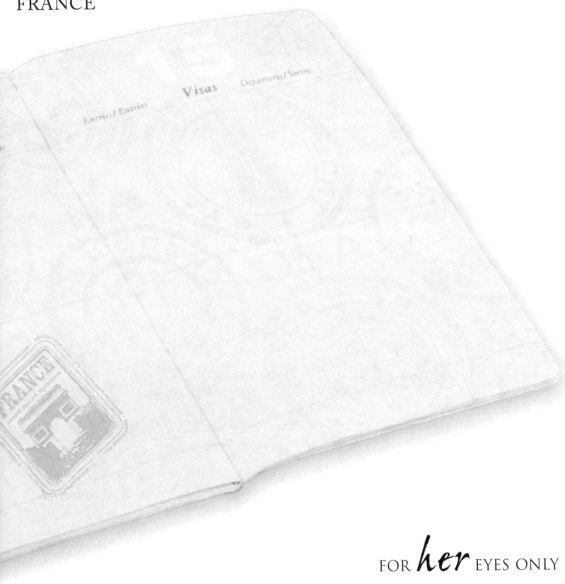

FOR *her* EYES ONLY

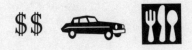

though. Frenchwomen are perfectly happy to wear wonderful lingerie like this under pretty daytime dresses or sundresses. As you go about your errands, you will discover the thrill that every *jolie jeune fille* knows. When you dress well, men notice. You'll feel their eyes on you. You'll see their smiles and sense their appreciation. You will love the attention. And you'll dig the secret thrill of traveling around town with nothing under your skirt. *I see London, I see France, I see . . .* well, *no* underpants.

This is a seduction that requires really, really, *really* good food. It doesn't have to be French, but it should be awesome, whether you buy it from a good restaurant or make it at home. (This is a great time to try out a cooking class, by the way.) Set up a terrific meal at home. Candles, music, wine. Eat slowly, and I'll bet you both will eat less. When you get up, every click of your high heels will remind him of what you have in store.

When you sit, call attention to your legs. Hike your hem and show off the tops of your stockings at the table.

Finally, move the action to your bedroom. Bring the candles. Set them all around you, like a halo of flickering light, so that you will be literally glowing as you unzip, unbutton, and undress for your man. Keep the lingerie on, of course. Climb on and make love the French way. *Lentement. Passionnément.*

Slowly. Passionately. *Et avec du chocolat!*

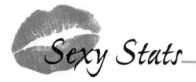

Sexy Stats

- Lingerie is *so* important to a Frenchwoman's sexual self-esteem that it comes as no surprise that only 3 percent of Frenchwomen see themselves as seductive when they're in the nude.

- If you're wondering *where* to spray your perfume before you dash out of the house, take some advice from famed designer Coco Chanel, who said when asked that question, "Wherever you want to be kissed."

- What item of lingerie turns men on the most? A whopping 80 percent of men in a survey on sexual weapons declared the garter belt to be their number one choice.

- Way back when, Cecil B. De Mille was directing a movie. A young actress was schlepping across the stage. De Mille told her tomorrow to wear sexy undies. "But Mr. DeMille," she said, "no one will know I'm wearing them." He responded, "No, but you will."

No. 24 HEART STRINGS

INGREDIENTS

2 stockings
2 high heels
2 exquisite meals

1 garter belt
1 pretty dress
many candles

THIS WEEK YOU'RE GOING TO HAVE FUN, EAT well, drive your man wild with lust, and . . . lose weight.

Sounds crazy, *non*? Ah, but *les femmes de la France* do it all the time, quite naturally, and so will you, once you see how easy and exciting it is. Your seduction begins, as do so many French activities, with lingerie.

Frenchwomen spend a lot on lingerie, almost 20 percent of their clothing budget, the most of all women in the Western world. Why? It's not just for seduction. (They are legendary for looking good in the boudoir, though.) After all, most of the time, no one sees what they're hiding under their work clothes. Which begs the question: Are French women so famously self-confident because of their sexy underwear . . . or do they wear expensive lingerie because they are confident?

Here's another question that people have been wrestling with. *How come they don't get fat?* The *salopes chanceuses*—and please don't ask your child to translate that for you; it's not polite!—get to eat French food their whole lives, with cream and butter and pastry and bread, and they stay amazingly slim. Scientists think they have an answer for that, which I don't pretend to understand. But I like what Mireille Guiliano says in her book called, you guessed it, *French Women Don't Get Fat*. Her theory is that the French simply take their time. A good meal is to be enjoyed slowly, with conversation

and laughter. Their food is rich, but they feel full before they've been able to eat too much of it.

That's a beautiful idea. And probably true. But here's Laura Corn's theory; *You can't eat much when you're wearing a garter belt*. It's a little snug around the middle. Go buy yourself a fantastic new garter belt and stockings. New heels, if you want. A matching bra is a plus. But you don't need a thong. (A *string*, it's called *en français*, and isn't that a perfect name for it?) You're going to be fashionable and gloriously free under your dress. *Haute* commando.

Show them to your guy when you get them home. Let him see how excited you are as you pull them out of your shopping bag. *"Oh, honey, aren't these gorgeous! So sexy! I can't wait to try them on for you."* Rest assured, he cannot wait to see you try them on, either. But wait he must, because this is just a tease for later in the week. Leave them out in the open, somewhere in the bedroom, so he can see them and think about them every day. Once or twice before bed, hold them up to you, over your clothes, and let him see how happy you are. Ask if he wants you to wear them, and when he says yes (or "duh!"), tell him too bad, he just has to wait a little longer. *Anticipation* means the same thing in French as in English.

Saturday morning, get dressed in front of him. Let him see you pull on the belt and stockings, and then hide it all under a flattering dress. You're not going for a cocktail party look,

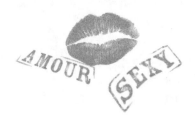
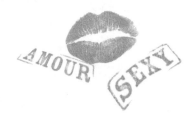
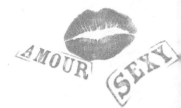
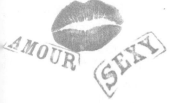
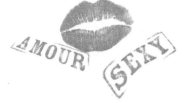
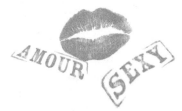
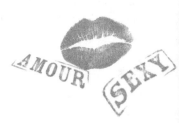
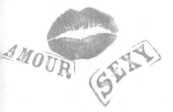
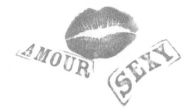
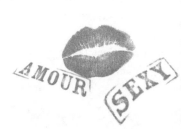

seduction no. 25

Stuck On You

GREAT BRITAIN

FOR *her* EYES ONLY

$

and undress him and get him warmed up, and then . . . tie his hands behind his back.

Uh-huh, you guessed it. Use the bondage tape around his wrists to make him horny and helpless. Sit him down and give him a good show as you take him into your mouth, hard and deep. But don't finish him. Instead, slowly ease off, backing away until your lips barely touch the tip. He'll be aching to push deeper. He'll want to put his hands on your head and take control, but *too bad!* No hands!

Move to a chair and spread your legs wide open. Tell him it's your turn and watch how he struggles to get to your cling-wrapped kitty using nothing but his tongue and teeth. You can help him, of course, slowly pulling away that final layer of transparent pink plastic between him and your waiting clitoris. Take your time here. Enjoy his oral skills. You can bet that he's enjoying a wicked little fantasy: bound and forced to service a woman.

Have him sit on the edge of the bed. Get him hard again with your mouth, and this time use lots of saliva, making sure his erection is completely wet. Now stand up, turn around, and sit in his lap. Wiggle and shimmy. *Wow.* You're creating an extraordinary, mind-boggling sensation for him, one he may never have felt before. The smooth plastic wrap, so snug across your bottom, is slipping and sliding against his wet shaft. It's sexy, and so *different*: slipperier than fabric, slicker than a condom, cooler and firmer than skin, softer and wetter than any hand. There are some wrinkles in the smooth surface of your skirt, and they tickle as they glide over his erection. It's crazy hot, and it makes him want to reach around and grab you, but of course, he can't. No hands, Bondage Boy!

Stay seated on his lap but slowly lift your pink skirt while you shimmy. He can feel the plastic sliding up. He can sense that the real thing, the thing he's dying for, the warm enveloping goodness of a woman's sex, is almost there, almost unveiled, and finally . . . *pop* . . . the barrier is breached. Now he feels your warm cheeks against his erection. In one quick move, you grab it and slide it inside you. *Ahhh.* Yes. Now he feels heat, and a different kind of wetness, and that lovely all-encompassing velvet squeeze that men were born to crave. This is the Queen's Position, and like her majesty, you are in complete control. Your subject is helpless and can do nothing but enjoy the sensation—and the awesome view— as you ride him to paradise.

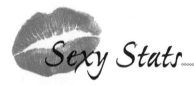 *Sexy Stats*

- The interrogation scene where Daniel Craig is tied to a chair in the James Bond film *Casino Royale* is one of the best-loved scenes by women everywhere.

- Madonna's 1993 book *Sex* depicted couples in bondage gear. In 2008, she gave another nod to bondage wear with a *Vanity Fair* pictorial.

No. 25 STUCK ON YOU

INGREDIENTS
1 or more rolls of plastic bondage tape, preferably in passionate pink
1 felt-tip marker

I LEARNED A PAINFUL LESSON SEVERAL YEARS ago.

Naturally, I'm always on the lookout for fun new bedroom tricks to share with readers, and that's how my misadventure started. I was trying to find a cute way to get a man's attention, and it hit me—guys just *love* duct tape. They fix stuff with it, they talk about it, and someone even wrote a book about it. And I thought, hey, wouldn't a guy think it was adorable and sexy and funny if I somehow used duct tape to seduce him? I was right. My guy *did* love the seduction. But sister, let me just warn you right now: If you get duct tape stuck on your skin, you had better be oiled up and shaved smooth.

Otherwise, *ouch*. Like getting an industrial-strength Brazilian wax. Like peeling off the world's biggest Band-Aid.

But that scariness is all in the past, because now there is—ta-da!—*bondage tape*. It's not really tape, not in the traditional sense, because it has no adhesive. It just sticks to itself and nothing else. In fact, it's really just cling wrap, like you might use to cover leftovers in your fridge, but it's available in narrower hand-sized rolls and it's, well, decorative. My first thought when I saw women wrapped in homemade pink tape miniskirts and tube tops on www.lovehoney.uk was, *"Wow!"* I was immediately inspired. Not only did it look sexy, but it looked like a fun thing to do. And it *was*!

It's always a good idea to grab a man's attention early in the week. Tear off short strips of the tape and leave them where he can't miss them, wrapped around the headrest of his car, for instance, or binding together his favorite shoes. As the weekend gets closer, crank up his sense of anticipation. Use a felt-tip marker to write a time and date on some of the tape: *Saturday, 7 P.M.* Each plastic note is a sweet little tease, and each one will put a smile on his face and remind him of you.

You need just the right outfit for this date, of course. And that outfit is . . . *pink bondage tape.* Yes, you're going to dress for sex-cess, entirely in pink plastic. Run a little pink strip between your thighs, like a thong, then make a tiny skirt by wrapping the pink plastic around your hips several times. Run the tape around your chest. And push your boobies up *high*. This stuff can give you super-cleavage.

Oh, you will have so much fun with this part of your seduction, making armbands and anklets and "jewelry" out of pink plastic. (And unlike the old gray duct tape, it comes off so easily! My pain is your gain. You're welcome.) Your man will be totally turned on when he walks in and sees your clingy new outfit. You'll look outrageously sexy and fun. He'll want to run his hands all over you.

Ah, but that's where this seduction takes a twist. He can't touch you. *No hands.* Kiss him

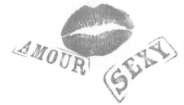
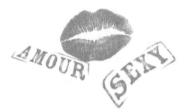
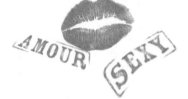
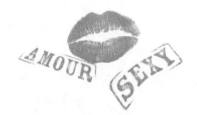

seduction no. 26

Room, Serviced

JAPAN

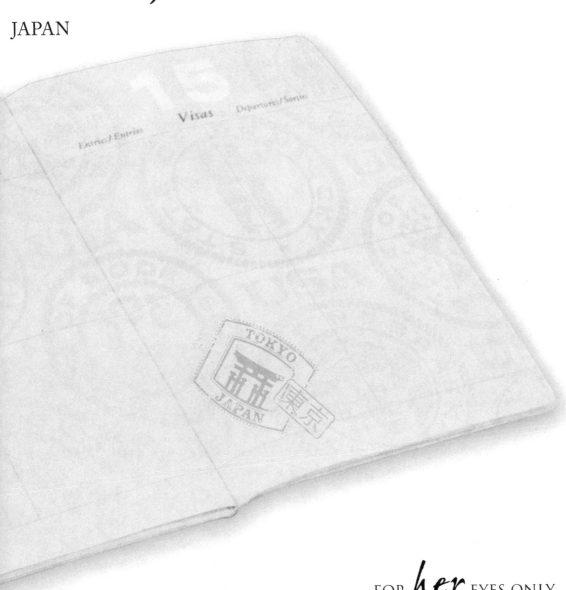

FOR *her* EYES ONLY

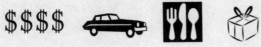

and lay them out. Now join your sweetie in the shower and stay there until you're both wrinkled and giggling. Lather each other up and dance around under the hot water. Kiss and slide and rub each other. Make him clean (and dirty) by gently washing his bat and balls, and slipping your soapy hands between his cheeks.

When he steps out of the bathroom and sees what you've done, he'll be totally amused, and totally impressed. On the bed, you've laid out two hypersexy outfits, and he gets to choose which one you will wear. One is some barely-there lingerie, and the other is the classic Japanese naughty-schoolgirl outfit, with over-the-knee white stockings and a plaid skirt. The linen-covered breakfast table now contains an assortment of sex toys and surprises, and he gets to pick his favorites for the morning. There's massage oil and lubricant. There's a vibrator or two. A silk scarf might be a blindfold, or it might be a bondage restraint. Bring whatever tickles your fancy. Nipple clips? Feathers? Penis jewelry? Temporary tattoos?

Be sure you bring some items purely for shock value. You might have no intention of actually using a giant strap-on dildo or Malibu Barbie, but wouldn't it be hilarious to see his reaction to them? The amenities you provide, and how far you *really* go over the next hour or two, all depend on your personal boundaries and how much you're willing to push them. And that is precisely the beauty of the Love Hotel. You can get as wild as you want, and maybe even a little wilder, and then go home as if it happened to two other people. Two people who happened to look like you, but were much less refined and dignified. Remember—

What happens in Osaka, *stays* in Osaka.

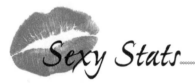

Sexy Stats

- Every day, around one million couples check into one of the nearly forty thousand *rabu hoterus*—love hotels—in Japan. Love Hotels are seen as mini–sex vacations, rented by the hour.

- Love Hotels come equipped with everything from vibrating beds to sunken baths, S&M equipment, and a selection of porno DVDs.

- A bonus at some of today's Love Hotels is the closed-circuit television system. Truly adventurous couples can watch other rooms, even as their own room is being watched.

- From free condoms at the Mercer Hotel in New York, to Sofitel's Lovers' Dice Game, to Mile High Kits available at upscale hotels like the W in Chicago and beyond, hotels are catching on that guests appreciate sex-themed amenities.

No. 26 ROOM, SERVICED

INGREDIENTS

1 hotel room with room service
2 sexy outfits
1 bottle personal lubricant
1 feather
assorted sex-related items, your choice (optional)
in-room adult video (optional)

1 breakfast in bed
1 vibrator
1 bottle massage oil
1 scarf
1 completely scary sex-related item (optional)

NOTE: If you have a no-children trip coming up in the near future, SAVE THIS SEDUCTION and use it in conjunction with your next hotel stay. Rip out a different seduction this week and keep this one in a safe place.

I DON'T KNOW IF THE WORLD WILL EVER BE ready for a huge Disneyland-style theme park devoted to the erotic arts. But if it does happen, I predict it will be built in Japan.

Why Japan? Because they are already halfway there. A combination of suppressed kink and limited real estate has created an extraordinary industry in The Land Of The Rising Sun. Every day, all over the country, amorous couples check into one of Japan's notorious Love Hotels. You can, if you wish, rent a room by the hour. But if you're picturing a seedy dive on the wrong side of the tracks, you're way off target. The Love Hotels of Japan are made for fun on an almost comical scale, like a tiny slice of the Vegas strip dropped into an otherwise quiet neighborhood. Some of the rooms have crazy themes and wild amenities. A giant Hello Kitty doll dressed in bondage gear. Bumper cars. Hanging basket chairs with holes in useful places. Vending machines filled with vibrators. A mock subway car, for those who get their thrills from the bump-and-grope of packed public spaces, but who prefer their *chikan* without incarceration.

There's even a Love Hotel with an old Cadillac convertible on the roof, and when guests set the car to rockin', the lights start flashing. Elvis would have *loved* this joint.

There's nothing quite like it in America. But with a little imagination and a credit card, you're going to create a Love Hotel experience that will have some huge long-term benefits—because your guy will be trying to top this one for the rest of his life.

Don't try to pull off this seduction on the night you check in. If you're like most couples, you'll be tired from traveling all day, and your guy may want to take you out to dinner. Instead, clear your calendar for a lazy morning in the room. Arrange for a late checkout. Best of all, splurge on room service breakfast. What decadence! The waiter rolls in a small table with white linen and china, as elegant as any fine restaurant. If you're a coffee drinker, getting a whiff of fresh brewed java *while you're still in bed* feels like a small peek into heaven. Food always tastes better when you're in your bathrobe, and better still if your room has a decent view. Breakfast in a hotel room is expensive and indulgent, but it can make two people fall in love all over again.

After your meal, tell your guy to hit the shower. While he's washing up, cover the empty plates and move them into the hall, but keep the breakfast table in the room. Bring out the seduction secrets you had hidden in your luggage

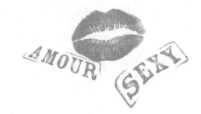
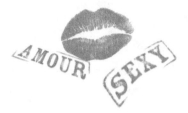
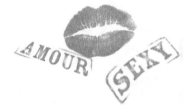

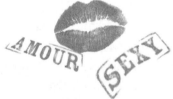
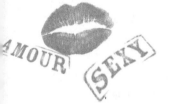
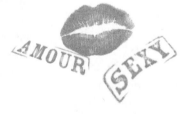
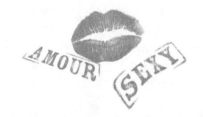
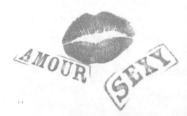

seduction no. 27

The Red Bandanna

MALIBU, CALIFORNIA, USA

FOR *his* EYES ONLY

sensuous thrill of fabric gliding across skin. They know, each and every one of them, the burning need to just be pinned back and taken by a mysterious man.

So here's your assignment this week. Get a cowboy bandanna and leave it in a place where your girl is bound to see it and wonder about it. Play with it a few times. Make her laugh. And then one night this week, tie it over your face like a bank robber . . . and get ready to steal her heart.

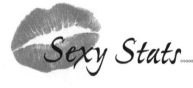 *Sexy Stats*

- Do women like it when men wear cologne? Worldwide, 92 percent say YES! (One of the most popular men's fragrances is Gucci's Envy.)

- Of the five senses—sight, hearing, touch, smell, and taste—smell has the most direct impact at an unconscious level. Smell affects one's mood and level of arousal by directly tapping in to the limbic system—that part of the brain that's involved with emotional behavior and memory.

- Bandanna is another name for kerchief. In Victorian times, kerchiefs were used as a means of flirtation. A woman could intentionally drop a dainty square of lacy or embroidered fabric to give a favored man a chance to pick it up as an excuse to speak to her while returning it.

No. 27 THE RED BANDANNA

INGREDIENTS

1 spray of cologne, gently applied
1 traditional cowboy-style bandanna
(Sure, you could probably use a Coach or Hermès scarf instead. You could wear mascara, too, and ask her to put highlights in your hair. But if you want to actually have sex, using your actual penis, it's best to stick with manly-man props. Cowboy up!)

I LOOKED ALL OVER THE WORLD FOR THE sexy tricks and tips that inspire the seductions in this book. Except for this one. This seduction is based on a true story that happened right in my own bedroom. It started as a joke, actually, a bit of silliness between Jeff and me. I was in bed after a long day and was, I confess, in no mood for love. Jeff started his cute prank, and—POW. Something amazing happened.

One moment I was giggling and pushing him away, and the next—I was hot. Smoking hot. He did something that shifted my mental image, and I found myself responding to him. The fantasy, the scent, the awesome masculinity of his move—it all worked some magic. And trust me when I tell you that this seduction has the power to take your woman from zero to 60 in three seconds flat.

It all started when Jeff came home after having a cigar with some buddies. I'll never say no to a kiss, but I laughed at this one and mentioned his breath, heavy with the smell of old tobacco. He went off to get ready for bed (and brush his teeth!), and when he came back, he was wearing a Red Bandanna across his face. He looked like a bank robber out of an old Western movie. He had the ends tied behind his head, with a triangle of fabric falling free over his nose and mouth. Just a joke. A token effort to keep his cigar breath from bothering me. But then he kissed me . . . and oh. My. GOD.

That one little layer of fabric across his lips made this kiss feel different from all other kisses. It was soft, and the softness of it slid across my lips every time he adjusted for a fresh kiss. The heat of his breath was trapped by the fabric, slowed enough that I became hyper aware of it—steamy, yummy heat hovering over my mouth, mixing with the warmth of my own lips, cooled only slightly by the red cloth.

I could smell something on the cloth, too, something delicious—oh, yes, he had put a dab of his cologne on it. I wasn't laughing now. I was making out, hard, and I found myself getting lost in the fantasy of it all. Later, I realized what had taken over my imagination. It's something I teach couples about, something I've talked about on the radio for years. Among women, the two most powerful, popular sexual fantasies are

1. Letting the man take charge, and
2. Sex with a stranger.

And here I was, getting surprisingly caught up in both fantasies at the same time. And when I say "caught up," what I really mean is that I was getting completely aroused and quickly heading for my first panty-soaking orgasm of the night.

Not, I am pleased to say, my last.

I've since told lots of women about The Red Bandanna, and they all *loved* it. They got it immediately. Women totally understand the power of scent, the erotic drama of a mask, the

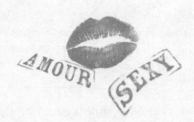

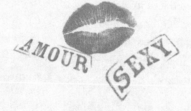
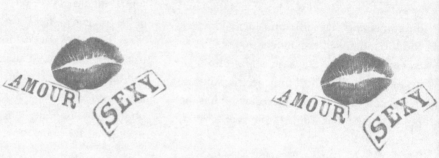
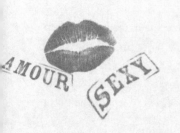

seduction no. **28**

Randy Roll

SOUTH AFRICA

FOR *her* EYES ONLY

not with you attached at the hip. Lock your legs onto him. Try to keep him from flipping you and rolling with you across the floor, because if he does, you are going to get wet, and not just between your knees. If he's a lot bigger than you, then you need to invoke one of the other rules of Naked Wrestling: No hands! *His* hands, that is; it's only fair.

Back and forth you go, rolling and wrestling, laughing and kissing, and making love hard all the while. In the end, it really doesn't matter who ends up on top, since you both get an orgasm if you win. And if you lose . . .

Well, how about that. You also get an orgasm, even if you've been licked. *Especially* then.

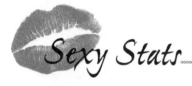

Sexy Stats

- Charlize Theron was not the first South African actress to be successful in Hollywood. Glynis Johns, who played the "Votes for Women!" suffragette mother in *Mary Poppins*, was born in Pretoria.

- "Theron" is pronounced "thrown" in Afrikaans. Think about that when you're channeling your inner South African naked wrestler.

- Boxing and wrestling are popular sports, for boys and girls, and the women's national wrestling team consistently does well in competitions. No wonder South African women are so tough!

No. 28 RANDY ROLL

INGREDIENTS
1 large space
1 blanket or sheet
candles
pillows
2 drinks (clear, nonstaining)

WHAT'S BEAUTIFUL, SPARKLING, BRILLIANT, multifaceted, and comes from South Africa? No, it's not a gemstone; I'm talking about a South African woman. The women of South Africa have struggled for gender equality for years, while remaining dignified, gracious, and strong. In recent years young women have excelled globally in sports, science, and technology. Academy Award winner Charlize Theron is probably the most famous South African in the world today, and in 2007 she was named the Sexiest Woman Alive by *Esquire* magazine. This week's seduction is based on the Randy Wrestling Roll from her native South Africa but with an all-American Laura Corn twist.

The morning of your seduction, call your guy into the living room and tell him you need some help pushing the furniture around. When he asks why, look him in the eye and tell him the truth. *"Because we're going to have sex there tonight, and I want to have some more room."*

Your man's brain is now boggled, and he'll spend the rest of the day with a grin on his face and a bulge in his shorts. When he meets you at home again, he'll see your living room decked out with candles, a blanket, a couple of drinks, and pillows—and he'll see *you* in a T-shirt and panties. Don't be coy. Tell him to hit the shower and get back out here. Don't shortchange the foreplay. You're a kick-ass woman tonight, and you should get all the action you want. He'll be happy to provide it, too, because almost every man has a secret *woman-in-charge* fantasy.

Here's where the game really starts. At some point, when he's deep inside you, tell him you're suddenly incredibly thirsty. You need to reach your drink, over across the room. *"But stay inside me. It feels soooooo good, just keep it inside, we can reach my glass."* Now roll with him, still coupled. And be ready to laugh, because, well, it's funny. (And challenging! Just wait until you try it.) Make sure you wind up on top before you grab your drink and take a sip. And then, with a sly smile on your face, reach into your glass, get your fingers wet, and flick your drink on his face. And just try to stay on top.

It will be like riding the world's sexiest bull in a rodeo. Laugh and flick some more drops on him. He will so want to flip you over and take revenge, but do your best to keep him trapped beneath you. Let him see a different expression emerge on your face, one that shows how much this wild ride is truly and totally turning you on. Put your glass down. *"Okay,"* you say again, *"but stay inside me."*

Now go for another roll. Let him spin you around. Spin him back, if you can. If he reaches for your drink to get a little revenge, tell him, uh-uh, that one's yours, and the rules of Naked Wrestling say that if he wants to get his own drink, well, it's all the way across the room . . . and you don't think he can get there,

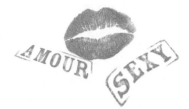
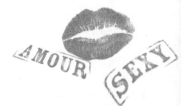
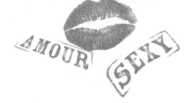

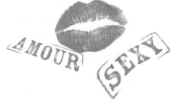

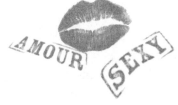
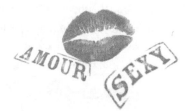
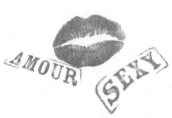

seduction no. 29

Breathe Me

INDIA

FOR *his* EYES ONLY

bedroom: *"Honey, let's breathe together for fifteen minutes . . ."* When she sees the scene you've set for her—the candles, the incense, the music playing softly—she won't be able to drop her towel fast enough! Go through the positions in order, staying in each one for five minutes.

POSITION 1: LEAN ON ME

Lead her to the bed, drop your towels, and sit with your back propped against the headboard with some pillows, legs apart. Have her sit between your legs and relax with her back on your chest. Now start synchronizing your breathing. Inhale the smell of her skin and hair as she leans into your chest, feeling your heartbeat.

POSITION 2: SPOON ME, BABY

Move down so that you're spooning together on the mattress with her body in front of yours, her body still snuggled into your chest. Continue to breathe together, and move your hips in rhythm with your breath. Your erection is pressed against her and can slide right between her thighs. So *close*, so *tempting*, but you're still building up to the main event. Stay five minutes here, keeping your breaths together, gently stroking her shoulders, caressing her breasts, and resting your hand over her mound as you move your hips in unison.

POSITION 3: LOVE IN LEGOLAND

Now you're feeling energized, your buddha is awake and excited, and you're ready for five minutes of penetration. Sit against the headboard with pillows behind your back. With your feet on the mattress, legs apart, pull her into your lap facing you. Put her hands behind your neck and guide your shaft into her. *Nice.* And *deep.*

Don't move. Hold your lover in your lap, wrap your arms around each other, and take a moment to get used to the feeling. You're stuck together like Legos now; there is no space between your bodies. You're holding her securely, and the feeling of weightlessness she gets is incredible, trust me. Take a few breaths together, face-to-face.

Then start to slowly rock yourselves back and forth. Your penis rubs against her G-spot, while your pubic bone gives her clit something to grind against—a magical combination when it comes to female orgasms. It may be a new sensation for your penis to be pulled in different directions while inside her. Enjoy it—and her response. The deeper your breathing, the easier it is to relax and let your orgasms rush through your bodies, exploding into a million stars above your heads.

Who's up for a yoga class?

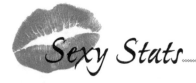

Sexy Stats

- Tantric sex practices have been around for seven thousand years. That's a lot of awesome sex!

- Kundalini is the name of an energy force—in the form of a serpent—that lies coiled at the base of the spine. According to Tantra, during orgasm, it is released and spirals up the spine.

- Most men are able to last longer if they've masturbated recently. This means that servicing yourself all week is good for her, too!

- The longest human orgasm recorded is 43 seconds. If you don't think that's impressive, sit in your chair and count to 43.

No. 29 BREATHE ME

INGREDIENTS
candles
incense
1 sheer scarf
relaxation sounds CD

IF YOU EXPERIENCE AN ERECTION LASTING LONGER than four hours . . ."

. . . Call your buddies and tell them how! Seriously, though, what if I told you there are men who *can* last that long, and without any little blue pills? And, no surprise, their partners are *very* happy.

Rocker Sting and his wife, Trudi, are probably the most famous couple singing the praises of Tantric sex and a rigorous Tantric yoga practice. If your sweetie or any one of her friends watches *Oprah*, I guarantee you she's heard about the amazing sex life of Sting and Trudi, and wants some of *that*. And what guy wouldn't want the stamina of that fifty-something dude?

Tantra takes years to master, but you can relax; I'm not sending you to yoga class . . . yet. This week I'm going to teach you a five-minute breathing technique that is virtually guaranteed to give you and your lover the orgasms of the century, no little blue pills required.

It's simple: *Breathe in and out through your nose.* Try it now, by yourself. You automatically have to breathe more slowly and controlled, right? You breathe more deeply. Hey, look at that, you're already more relaxed. Keep breathing like that for five minutes. That's it.

That's it? Yes, but it takes two to tango (or, in this case, to yab-yum), and you need a partner. This week you're going to practice that breathing technique in *three different sexual positions* with

your girl. In fifteen minutes, your neighbors could be wishing for earplugs.

Titillate your sweetheart each day with a link to a video or an article at www.tantra.com. Make sure to send her an article on the definition of Tantra, one about breathing (there are several) and one or two different techniques you're interested in. She'll definitely be intrigued and will take a peek around for herself. Keep it *simple*; this seduction is to give you both a taste of Tantra and whet your appetites for more.

On Friday send her an e-mail from work: *I've been really getting into this Tantra stuff. What do you say we practice Tantric breathing together? Tomorrow at 9?* She'll be flabbergasted and more than ready for your exotic seduction.

Here's how *you* get ready:
* Take a shower (women love a clean man).
* Draw her a bath with her favorite bath oil (or try a few drops of Nag Champa oil; its exotic, peppery scent is *made* for deep inhalations).
* Change the sheets while she's bathing.
* Light a few candles in the bedroom.
* Burn some incense to create an exotic atmosphere.
* Drape a scarf over the lampshade.
* Put on some mood music (try Ravi Shankar or a Hearts of Space CD).

When she's done with her bath, meet her in the bathroom wearing a towel and wrap her in one. Take her hand and lead her into the

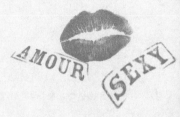

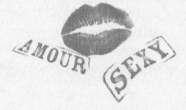

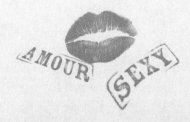
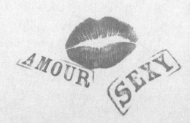

seduction no. 30

CINQ À SEPT

FRANCE

FOR *his* EYES ONLY

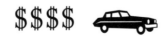

to the room, change, and meet me in the bar at six.
Amazing. Awesome. Thrilling!

There, on the bed, is her whole outfit, neatly laid out. (Killer option, if you want to spend a little more money: *a wig*. It's the turbocharger under the hood of every woman's fantasy.) She'll freshen up, put on her clothes, check herself in the mirror, and feel *hot*. She'll know that every eye is on her when she strolls into the bar. It's a gorgeous bar, and your expression assures her that you think she is the most gorgeous thing in it. Flirt with her. Make her feel desired.

Everything you're doing has a purpose. The surprise date, the elegant bar, the outfit, and the hotel room all help to transform her into a different woman. They separate her from her stressful workday life and let her become a lover, a fantasy . . . a mistress. The French are famously tolerant of *petites amies*, little loves on the side, and they love those magic hours—*cinq à sept*,

five to seven—when anything goes. But you have something better. You have your true love *and* your crazy fling, and no need to hide one from the other. You get the best of both. All you really needed to do was remind your girl that she could *be* both.

And at the moment, she is in wildly sexual mistress mode. So finish that drink and get back to your room. Pin her to the wall and kiss her hard. Ravish her. Remove just enough of her *très chic* outfit to give her the *real* French kiss. (And in French, the word is . . . *cunnilingus*! Don't worry about the rest of her clothing yet; there's plenty of time to remove that before round *deux*. Oh, yes, there will be a second round, and maybe a third, thanks to another important lesson in this seduction, one that works as well in Poughkeepsie as in Paris:

The best sex is hotel sex.

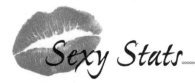

Sexy Stats

- In France, *cinq à sept* means time for fooling around. In the old days, a Frenchman could see his mistress at five and be home for dinner by seven, no questions asked. These days, though, the French are more likely to have their *cinq à sept* from two to four. Why? Traffic jams. Can't get off, or get anywhere, at 5 P.M.

- Stateside, upscale hotels like W offer "Pleasure Packages" and "Intimacy Kits" (with sex toys!) for their guests. Kudos to hotels for recognizing that yes, people do like to have sex in their rooms.

- In French culture, the *non dits*—the things you *don't* say—are just as important as the things you do say. Leaving a little unsaid creates mystery and lights the fires of passion.

- The city of Paris has well over 2,000 hotels.

No. 30 CINQ À SEPT

INGREDIENTS
1 elegant hotel with a beautiful bar
1 suitcase

How would you like some hot, adventurous sex?

Better yet, what if this sex was with a happy, carefree woman who adores you and thinks that you hung the moon? A lascivious woman who will gleefully, um, *do things* to you? And even better—what if this great sex actually had a lasting positive effect on your home life?

It's surprisingly easy. Just get a mistress.

Kidding! What I really mean is, every once in a while, you should treat your mate as if she were your mistress. Court her. Seduce her in grand style. Take your partner out of her normal routine and put her in a place where she is your crush, your centerfold, your *objet du désir*, your fantasy girl. It's not a place where she might want to live all the time—who could get any work done, with all that adoration going on?—but she'll love visiting there. And she'll reward you for arranging the trip. Some of your reward will be obvious, of course: She'll be your *petite minette sexy*, your little sex kitten, and she will pleasure you until you are *sore*. Seriously, you should probably limber up before the weekend.

The bigger impact of this seduction will come in the days and weeks afterward. When you go big, when you swing for the fences like this, you are actually *erasing her doubts*. She can't help but have them, you know. Every woman eventually starts to wonder if her guy still finds her attractive. This seduction washes away those concerns. A big display of passion like this boosts her confidence, which makes her a better lover. It makes her happier, which makes her a better partner in all other aspects of life. In short—it greases the gears of your relationship.

Think of it like maintenance on your car. Expensive, maybe, but nothing compared to the cost of *not* doing it.

Begin your seduction with a startling request. Early in the week, ask her to put together a favorite out-on-the-town outfit, something she likes to be seen in. The whole thing: dress, lingerie, shoes, stockings, whatever. Tell her to leave it on the bed by Thursday, because *you have a plan*, and that's all she needs to know. Tease her with that phrase all week. *"I have a plan for you!"* Speak it, text it, e-mail it. It will make her crazy. You'll be the talk of her girlfriends.

Thursday, gently fold her outfit into a small suitcase, then toss it into your trunk. She will, of course, be buzzing with anticipation, but the only thing you can tell her is, *"Tomorrow afternoon; instructions to follow; watch for e-mail."*

After a day of dancing on the Get Mail button, I'll bet she gasps when your message finally shows up. *5:00, front desk of the Hilton Hotel on Broadway—the clerk has something for you.* Wow. Cool.

When she gets there, the man at the desk hands her an envelope. It holds a key and a note: *Go*

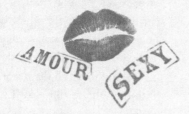

seduction no. *31*

You Might Feel a Little Prick

GREAT BRITAIN

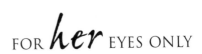

FOR *her* EYES ONLY

$$

You can put his mind at ease; it's not that kind of exam. Or . . . *is* it?

No, the gloves and the lube are for another kind of test. Check him out for what the medical professionals call *erectile dysfunction*. And what your lover will remember as *the best hand job of his life*. You've stroked him before, but now the smooth latex, the copious amounts of lubricant, the wicked fantasy costume all add up to an extraordinarily erotic experience for him. Throw a pillow down so you can kneel at his bedside. Encourage him to slip his hand under your skirt so he can play with your neatly trimmed bits. Kiss him while you slide your slippery fingers up and down, up and down, slowly building up speed and pressure until you feel his back arch and body tremble.

This is one medical bill he won't mind paying.

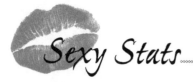

Sexy Stats

- It's a fact: Having sex the same way repeatedly gets boring. It actually changes our brain chemistry! Role playing wakes up the imagination, making sex new and exciting again. Sometimes, choosing to be someone as different from ourselves as possible is the best medicine against boring sex.

- Naughty Nurse costume is the number one dress-up fantasy for guys.

- Guess who else likes to give sponge baths to their patients, I mean, partners? Christina Aguilera (who bought her hubby a doctor costume so they could play hide the stethoscope), Carrie Bradshaw, a few desperate housewives, and Kate Moss just to name a few.

- Wondering where to discreetly buy a fantasy nurse costume? www.3wishes.com carries more varieties than you can shake a thermometer at.

No. 31 YOU MIGHT FEEL A LITTLE PRICK

INGREDIENTS
1 sexy nurse costume
1 pair latex gloves
1 bottle personal adult lubricant
sex toys (optional)

IT WAS A TOUGH CALL, BUT IN THE END I HAD to credit this seduction to Great Britain. But not because of British men. They are just as gobsmacked by the Naughty Nurse fantasy as every other man in the Western world. I might change my mind, though. If the Heart Attack Grill in Arizona ever goes nationwide, then this fantasy will definitely fall back into the America column. The Grill is a place where the fries are cooked in pure lard, the burgers can be stacked four artery-clogging patties high, and the waitresses are dressed in, you guessed it, smoking-hot fantasy nurse costumes.

Real nurses are not amused. Personal-injury lawyers are licking their chops, though.

Here's why the UK gets to claim this fantasy: It's the women. The birds, man! They understand that sex may be important, but it shouldn't be *serious*. English girls are masters of erotic dress-up. They buy these fabulous outfits and costumes to turn on their guys, and they are clearly having a bloody good time themselves. A consistent British favorite is the Naughty Nurse, two generations after real nurses switched to unglamorous scrubs.

No big anticipation teasers this week. Costume play is often best when it's a surprise. (Though the usual rules of surprise sex apply: no kids underfoot, no championship game on the tube, no beans for dinner. It's for your own good.) Saturday evening, casually mention that you have a new outfit you want your guy to see. Bring it up a few times during dinner. Make him promise that he'll give you his opinion about it when you model it later. Finally, send him to bed a little early, then slip into the bathroom to put on your costume.

The basic vinyl Naughty Nurse dress is cheeky and inexpensive, but if your budget allows, you can really dress it up with matching shoes and thigh-highs, sexy underwear, and a doctor's bag filled with sex toys. Call out to him to make sure he's ready for your entrance, and then . . .

Strut into the room on the tallest heels you own. *"Someone called for a sponge bath in this room?"* Va-va-va-VOOM! Real working nurses cringe at this stereotype, but this is no time for political correctness. *"Maybe I should check your chart."* Turn to face your dresser, with your back to your patient, and bend deeply enough to let him see your cheeks under your super-short white uniform. *"Are you comfortable today?"* Your underwired breasts spill into his face as you lean over to fluff his pillow.

Laugh, play, kiss. Have fun examining his body. And then watch his eyes bug out when you reach for the only actual medical gear you need for this seduction: latex gloves and a tube of K-Y Jelly. Feel him twitch when you *s-ss-ss-snap* the gloves on. Notice how his butt cheeks clench when you squirt the lubricant onto your fingers.

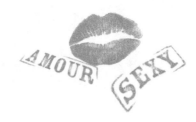
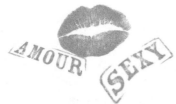
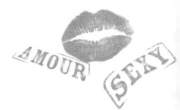
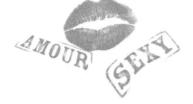
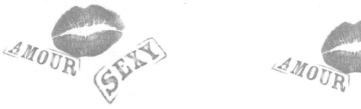
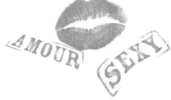
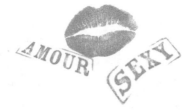

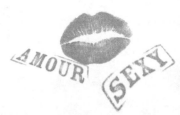

seduction no. 32

The Hot Herb Ball Massage

THAILAND

FOR *her* EYES ONLY

$$

a man between your thighs?) Reach for one of the warm, steamy herb balls and press it into his skin. Let the heat soak in before moving it to a different spot. Give him the hot treatment all along his spine, and especially on the hard, tense muscles of his neck.

Just when he's gotten used to the idea that you were talking about these cotton balls all along instead of, you know, the other ones, surprise him. Make him flip over. And show him a different kind of ball massage.

Test the heat of the herbal balls against your wrist before applying them to any of his sensitive bits. He might gasp at first. He'll definitely moan. The sensation of heat on his balls is astonishing and extraordinarily pleasurable. The warm, moist bundle of herbs reminds him of your mouth but even hotter. Wrap your lips around the top of his erection and show him your oral skills. Let him savor the warmth and the wonderful aromatherapy smell.

Now, straddle him again, this time with your back to him in the reverse cowgirl position. What a truly awesome view, for *both* of you—he gets to see your magnificent backside riding his hips; you get to see his shaft plunging in and out of you. His boys bounce between your thighs with pent-up energy. Reach for a couple of herb balls, test them for temperature, and then place them *right down there*—on his balls and on your clit. Pull them away and feel the chill as the wetness evaporates; put them back and let the heat soak in again. Repeat as desired.

You know what happens outdoors when heat meets cold. Crazy things start to happen with the weather. Hot and cold can do crazy things when they collide on your skin, too. Pleasure builds into rolling thunderheads. Erotic lightning fills the air.

Boom—it's storm season in your bedroom.

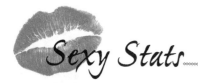

Sexy Stats

- In the film *Tomorrow Never Dies*, the debonair woman seducer, James Bond, was handcuffed to a beautiful Chinese spy as he raced through a Bangkok back alley on a motorcycle.

- More *yim* for your *yang*: the smile (*yim* in Thai) is so valued, it is rare to see an unhappy face on the streets of the country. The act of smiling increases dopamine, a natural antidepressant.

- Thai women are famous for their gracious hospitality and warmth. Their genial approach to life makes it clear why they're often the first contact visitors have with the country, and why so many men find them irresistible.

- Hot-stone massage kits, with stones, tongs, a warmer, and instructions, are available online. Warm stones are laid on the body, warming it and releasing tension. Sounds like the perfect prelude to an herb ball massage.

No. 32 THE HOT HERB BALL MASSAGE

INGREDIENTS

2 or more Thai herb balls (www.universaltouchinc.com)
1 Crock Pot, steamer, or bowl with hot plate
candles
massage oil

QUICK, WHAT DO YOU THINK WHEN I SAY HOT Herb Ball Massage?

You might be thinking about a ball stuffed with herbs, like a bag of potpourri. Or maybe you thought I meant hot *herbal* massage.

But say that to a guy, and all he hears is *ball massage*! And he's thinking, *Ooh, that might be really nice, if you don't squeeze them too hard.* Your sweet man may be too polite to say all that out loud, but I promise you he's thinking it. And that testosterone-driven confusion is what makes the Hot Herb Ball Massage the funniest thing you will ever see in Thailand. Male tourists stare at the menu in front of Thai massage parlors, pondering the meaning of the phrase and wondering just exactly what gets rubbed inside.

The truth is, a guy probably *could* get the twins tickled in Thailand as easily as he could anywhere else, if he found the right place. But the real Hot Herb Ball Massage is, in fact, an ancient massage technique that requires a special mixture of dried herbs that are wrapped in a cotton cloth and then tied into a ball. The original Thai recipe uses almost a dozen ingredients, which can be bought online, or you can create your own herb balls using those items. Either way, your house is going to smell heavenly. And when you do it the Laura Corn way, your man is going to get his happy ending, guaranteed. You, too.

Start by teasing your guy early in the week. *"Hey, honey, I ordered some stuff for a ball massage!"*

Wha—? You did *what*?

Don't explain. Just smile and tell him not to peek in the mail, because his balls could come any time. Ahem. As the weekend approaches, tease him some more. *"Gosh, I haven't seen your balls yet."* Thursday, send him an e-mail: *Ball massage tomorrow night. You should probably shave.*

Friday night, he'll smell an amazing aroma coming from your Crock Pot. The herbs inside the cotton-wrapped balls are steeping in hot water, releasing the pungent fragrances locked inside. Lemongrass . . . eucalyptus . . . safflower . . . tamarind—the scents fill the air and draw your guy over. *"It's the herb balls,"* you explain. *"For your herb ball massage."*

Oh, so that's what you meant. A massage with herb balls. Because I thought—never mind.

Ask him to carry the Crock Pot to the bedroom to keep his, um, balls warm. (You could also use a regular bowl and a hot plate.) Light candles and have him get undressed. Begin with a traditional massage—lots of oil, lots of pressure, lots of long loving strokes across his skin. Strip down to T-shirt and panties so you can straddle the small of his back while you work. (Mmm—don't you just love the feeling of

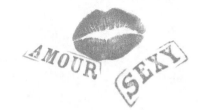
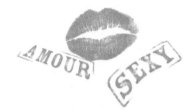
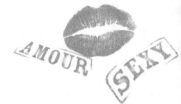
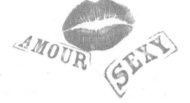
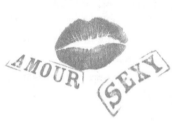

THE HOTTEST SEX FROM AROUND THE WORLD

seduction no. 33

Bodyrock

GREAT BRITAIN

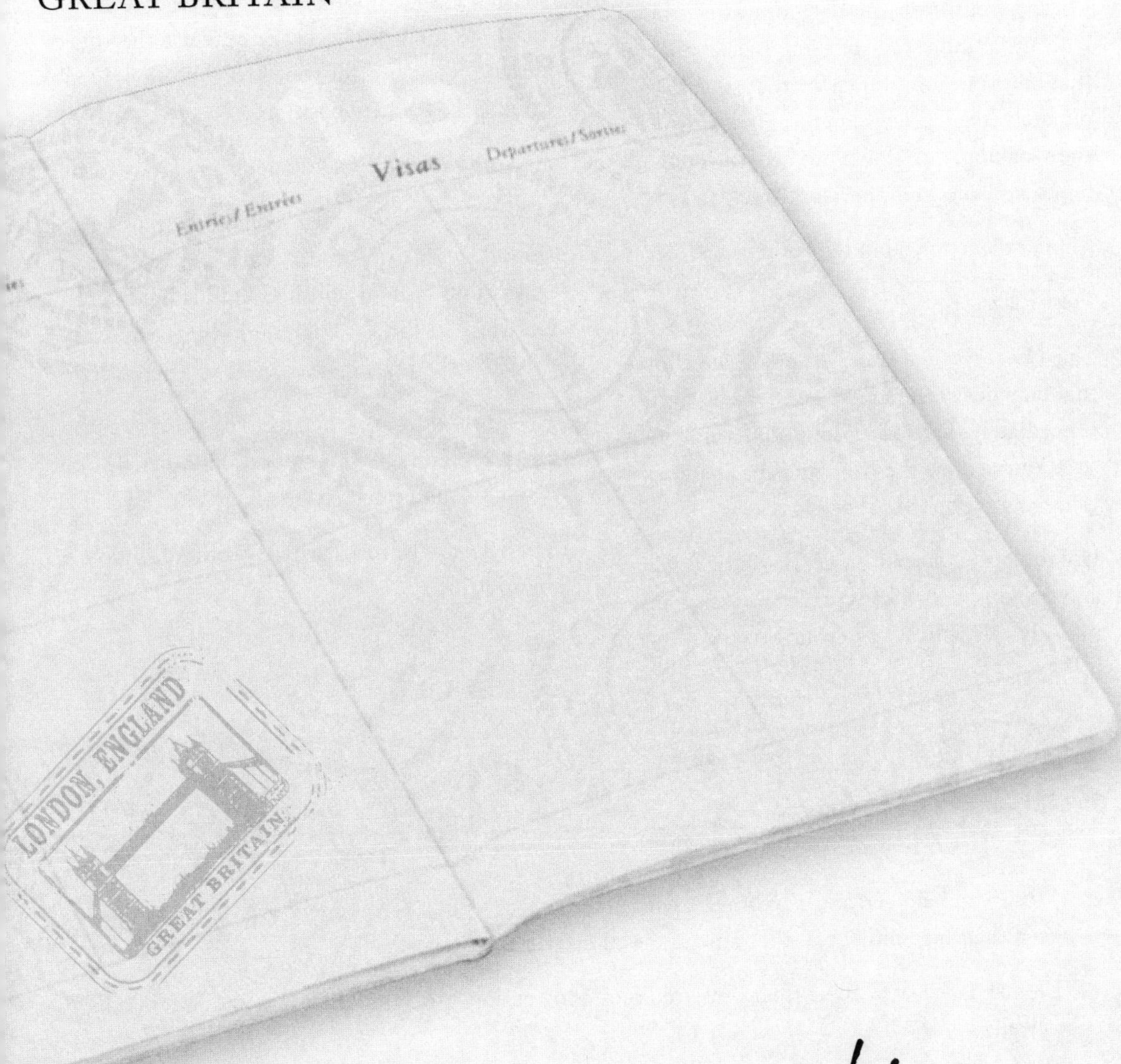

Visas
Entries/Entrées
Departures/Sorties
LONDON, ENGLAND
GREAT BRITAIN

FOR *his* EYES ONLY

choices for each "scene," and narrow the larger list down to a manageable size.

Download the songs, or go old school and make her a mix from CDs you already own. Once you have ten or so songs, you're ready to put it all together. The sound track should start out slow and easy, increase in speed and intensity, and wind slowly down.

On the evening of your date, draw her a bubble bath and put on some relaxing music: nothing that's on your sound track or that sounds remotely like it. Play something relaxing. While she's soaking, turn down the bed, turn down the lights, and cue your playlist to track 1.

Let her come to you in the bedroom.

Press Play.

She'll hear the first song—the one she chose that puts her in the mood—and she'll know immediately that you've done something very sexy. You've done the work and made something especially for her. That's *hot*.

Use the music as your guide. Begin by kissing and stroking her all over while the warm-up plays. It's all right to take your time; you've got a built-in formula and the music will be your cue to move on to the next scene. Increase the intensity gradually so it feels seamless to her. Hold her close while you kiss her and press your erection against her thigh.

Look at her: She's not thinking about library books or car pools: she is right here, with *you*. You're both hot now, the music is pulsing, and your bodies are finding their way together. Listen to the words, feel the beat, use the entire surface of the bed for your sexual healing. Don't hold back. Try new positions.

And when the beat starts pounding, start *rocking*.

When you've both collapsed and the music has slowed again, catch your breath and look at each other. Your faces are flushed, your skin is wet, and you just shook her all night long. So *that's* why it's called *afterglow*.

And from now on, whenever you want to cause a physical and emotional reaction in her, just put on your sound track.

You'll always be ready whenever that London fog rolls in.

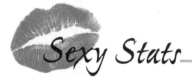

Sexy Stats

- Music can help get your rhythms in sync, according to a poll of women who say music helps keep their hips moving at the same rate as their partner's.

- English lads list R&B as their preferred music to get down to, but electronica and jazz rate high as well.

- Music tech, meet sex tech: The iBuzz is a vibrator you plug into your stereo or MP3 player. When the music speeds up, so do the vibrations.

- The sound track for the film *9 1/2 Weeks*, with sexy songs by Joe Cocker and Bryan Ferry, is an all-time hit with the ladies. Sticking "You Can Leave Your Hat On" in your sound track virtually guarantees that someone's going to take her clothes off.

INGREDIENTS
a mix CD or playlist
CD player or MP3 player and portable speakers

WHAT IF I TOLD YOU THAT YOU'RE NOT HAVING as much sex as you could be having?

Really, you're not, and here's why: British men have more sex annually than Americans, and the majority of them do it to music. Coincidence? I think not.

Men in Britain have caught on that *sex with a sound track* is sex worth remembering. Maybe it's because there's so much great music happening in the UK, or perhaps it's all that London fog making folks *randy*; doing it to music is one of the simplest ways to transport yourself and your lover to another place. Over the next few days, you're going to compile a sound track for your bedroom. And you're going to get your lady to help.

First, make a list of songs to make out to. (You had a sexy make-out tape in college, didn't you?) Your list should be around twenty songs long and include smooth songs, upbeat songs, hard pounding songs, and yes, love songs. This is a seduction, after all. The key to a good sound track is to tell a good story, with a beginning, a middle, and an end. A good sound track is also evocative. So much so that whenever you put on this mix, her heart speeds up, her knees go weak, and you *know* you're getting laid.

Divide your list into scenes. These songs are suggestions. You can choose your own, as long as you follow the formula:

KISSING & FOREPLAY
"Breathe Me" by Sia
"Bleeding Love" by Leona Lewis
"Sexual Healing" by Marvin Gaye

ORAL & SLOW LOVEMAKING
"Glory Box" by Portishead
"Ain't No Sunshine" by Bill Withers
"Every Breath You Take" by The Police

INTERCOURSE
"Radar Love" by Golden Earring
"Still of the Night" by Whitesnake
"You Shook Me All Night Long" by AC/DC

AFTERGLOW
"Porcelain" by Moby
"Wicked Game" by Chris Isaak

PILLOW TALK
"Each Coming Night" by Iron & Wine
"Arms of a Woman" by Amos Lee

Now you're ready to get your sweetie involved. It's going to take some preparation on your part, but when you're done you'll have a sex sound track that you can use again and again. Send her an e-mail one day with a few of the slower songs and a note: *Which of these puts you in the mood?* File her response, because it's the first song on your sound track. The next day, send another e-mail with another question: *Which of these songs makes you want to be kissed?* Follow that with: *These songs make me want to put my fingers inside you: Which do you like?* Keep giving her several

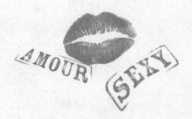
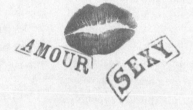

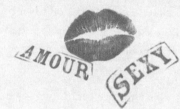
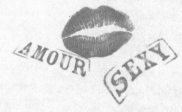
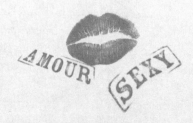
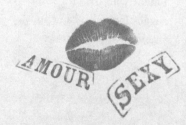

seduction no. 34

Seoul Sister

SOUTH KOREA

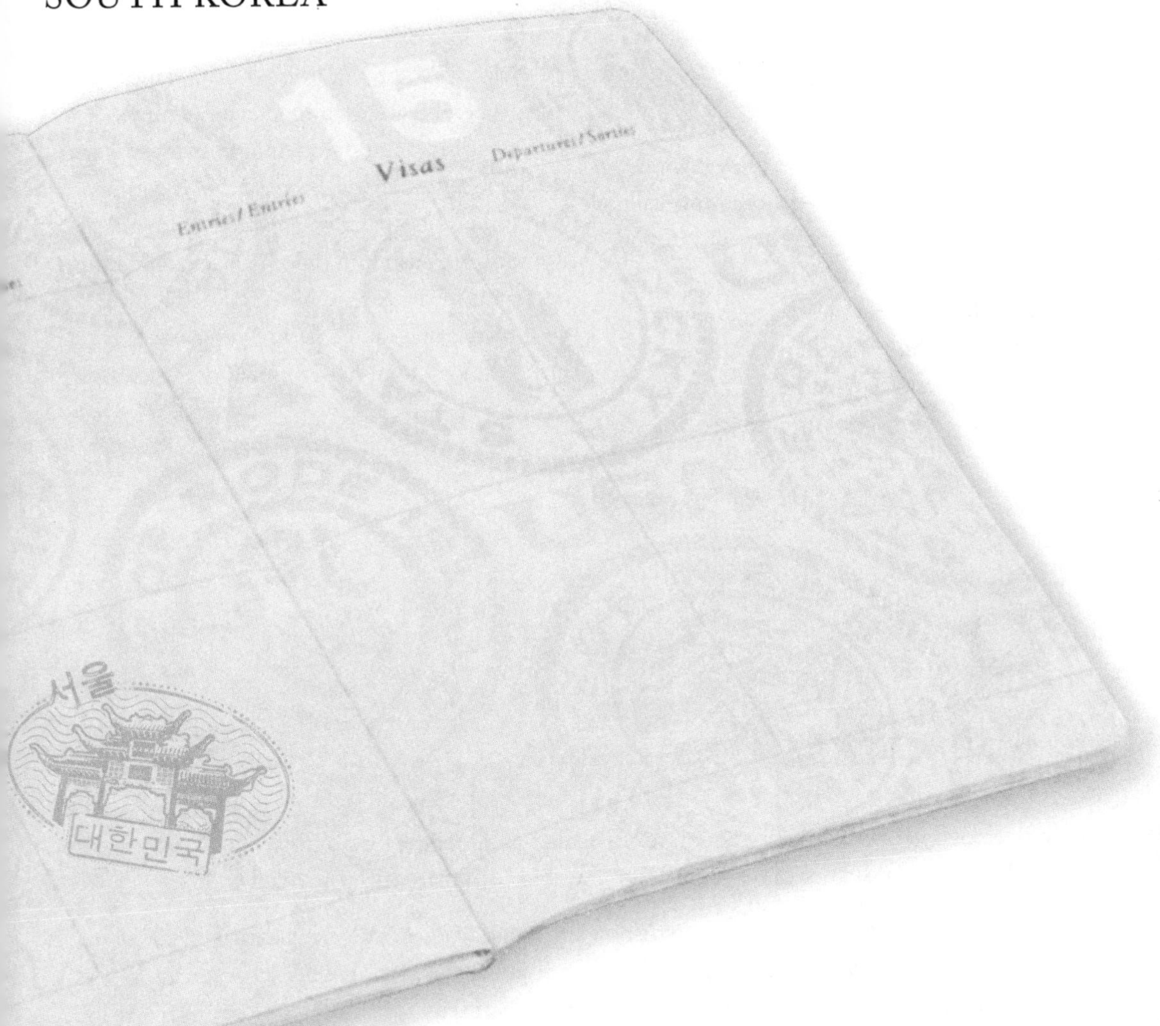

15

Visas   Departures/Sorties

Entries/Entrées

서울

대한민국

FOR *her* EYES ONLY

Then touch yourself for a moment, feeling how wet you are. Make him guess again what you're doing. Watch him harden right before your eyes as he strains to imagine.

You may want to pounce on him once you see how eager he is for you, but hold off. This is a sensual, teasing way to act out some light BDSM and give him the kind of pleasure he can get only from giving it up to you. Release him from his pants and feel how hard he is for you. Then take the other scarf and let it flutter against him.

"What do you want?" you can ask him, always keeping in mind that you are the one who will decide what he will get. Fasten the scarf around his balls—you can tie it into a knot, or just tug on it to give them a little squeeze before placing your hand around him. You aren't going to give him a hand job, because what he's got is for you to savor. You want to work him into a fervor, see how he reacts as you tighten the silk.

Use the scarf on his whole body, almost like a massage. Use it to tickle his neck, pinch his nipples through its fabric, blow on it so it caresses his skin. You can tie his wrists lightly together or for further penis play. The point is, in those moments, to channel those fierce South Korean women who know what they want and go after it. You're in charge. And he won't say a word in protest because he's at peak arousal.

Remind him of all that he can't see. Strip off your clothes so he can hear you, but dance away when he wants to touch you—unless you just can't stand the temptation any longer; then you're free to give him a taste. Keep the blindfold on him and when you're ready to mount him, push him onto his back and climb on top. It's time to give him a guided tour of your own erotic theme park. And you're in luck—he's brought his own phallus.

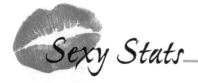

Sexy Stats

- Asian women know that their reaction to sex makes all the difference in their men's enthusiasm for it. Encourage a partner to try something new and then react enthusiastically.

- Dressing in costume and role playing isn't new for Asian women. Wigs, makeup, and elaborate costumes add to the characters, some of the most popular of which are sexy schoolgirl, dominatrix, geisha, and even prostitute, all in the name of fantasy.

- Love Land is also known as "Honeymoon Island" in South Korea, and serves as an impromptu sex ed class for newlyweds. Since many marriages are still arranged, couples might actually benefit from a climb up the thirty-foot-tall stone phallus.

No. 34 SEOUL SISTER

INGREDIENTS
2 silky scarves

WHO KNEW THAT SOUTH KOREA WAS A PLACE where men are having more sex than anywhere else in the world—four times a week? They also have a theme park called Love Land with a phallus garden and other explicit sculptures, the perfect setting for the true voyeur (or a hot date).

It's not all about the men, either. South Korean women aren't just passive participants. In a survey, 94 percent of them considered their sex life important. Wow! We can all learn a lesson from that. Privileging sex and making it a priority, thinking about it throughout the day, not just when the lights are out, can fuel your fantasies and make you eager to tear his clothes off when you see him again.

But before you do, wait a minute. Another area where these ladies are mistresses of their domain is in overpowering their men in the bedroom. As Kyung-Hae Yoon, editor of *Cosmo* in Korea, noted in an article regarding sex practices around the world, "Before the sex act even begins, [*Cosmo*] readers will blindfold their boyfriends with scarves and then tantalize them by slowly dragging silk over their bodies from head to toe, lingering extra long around his pelvis area."

So what does this mean for you and how can you get a little bit of that South Korean magic for yourself? All you need are two silky scarves, which you probably already have in your closet.

Now instead of adorning your neck, they're going to go somewhere much more intimate.

Using a scarf has a few pluses. One, you already have it in the house, so there's no need to buy something special. Two, it probably smells like you and will remind him of you as you use it to torment him. Its softness is alluring, and perhaps a bit deceptive, because you're going to use it to drive him to the edge of passion.

You don't have to act like a dominatrix to take charge. This is not about ordering him to do your bidding but convincing him that this is what he wants most in the world. Move gracefully as you take the scarves out of your dresser drawer. If he asks what they're for, tell him, *"You'll see."* Or rather, *not* see!

Let him touch the fabric that is going to be used to make him want you even more. Both of you can luxuriate in its slippery delight. Let it flutter between your legs, give a breathy sigh or giggle, then jokingly but firmly push him onto the bed, faceup. *"There are so many things I could do with this . . ."* you can tell him.

"Like what?" he'll ask as you run a hand from his balls on up until you're patting his cheek. Hint at what's to come, and he will be putty in your hands.

"Like this," you can say as the scarf is tied around his eyes. *"How many fingers am I holding up?"* Make him guess.

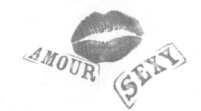

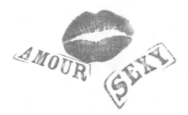

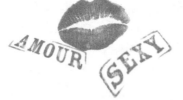

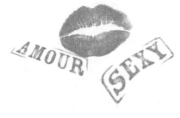

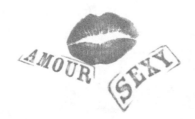

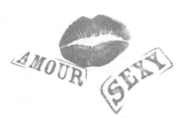

seduction no. 35

Sex & Candy

USA

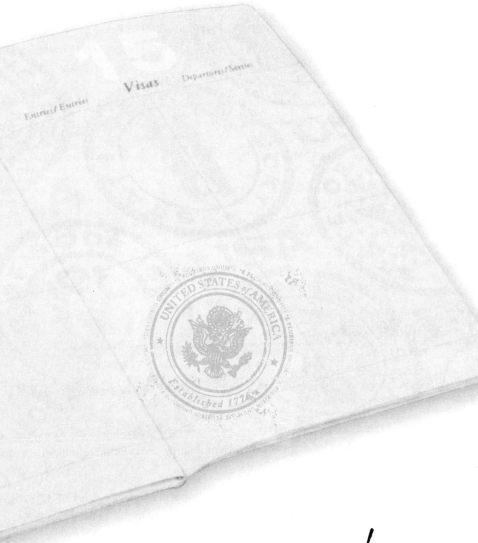

FOR *her* EYES ONLY

and suck it like . . . well, like it's *him*. Wink. Tell him to count to one hundred and then follow you to bed. One . . . two . . . three four fivesixseveneight*ninetynineonehundred*.

You've had time only to pull off your pants and climb onto a pile of pillows on the bed. But that's all you need, that and your sucker. Pull it out of your mouth. Slowly, dramatically, touch it to your thigh, just above your knee. *"Come here and lick this,"* you tell him, pointing to the sticky spot on your leg.

Yum! He'll be on the bed in a flash, nibbling the lolly-print. *"Good boy! Now . . . lick this."* Lift your leg and apply the lollipop to the back of your thigh. Enjoy the warmth of his tongue as he laps up your sugar. He gets it now. You press the pop somewhere, and he follows with his mouth. *Sweet!*

Touch it to your neck. Pull off your shirt and draw a line of sweet spots across your tummy. Use the lollipop to lead his tongue to your hips, your breasts, your mouth. Then turn the tables. Start applying the candy to *his* skin and following it with your tongue. Neck, shoulders, nipples (don't forget to lick his nipples—*wow!*) and, of course, take your time drawing sugary circles all around his stick. Ooh, yes, that's what he's been dreaming of all day. That's what he's been imagining, ever since you started teasing him. He's waiting for you to make his lolli—

Pop!

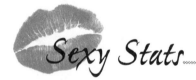

Sexy Stats

- In nearly every book or column about sex techniques, the Lollipop Lick is listed as one of the great oral techniques you can master.

- In 1916, a Russian immigrant was given the keys to the city of San Francisco for inventing a machine that inserted sticks into candy, thereby automating the creation of lollipops, and forever associating the City by the Bay with sucking.

- For maximum lolly inspiration, listen to "Candy Shop" by 50 Cent, "I Want Candy" by Bow Wow Wow, "Sex and Candy" by Marcy Playground, "Lollipop" by Lil Wayne, "Lollipop" by Mika, and of course, "Lollipop," by the Chordettes.

- Lollipop lick. Recall those long and twisty lollipops from the carnivals, the ones that you cannot possibly fit all the way into your mouth. So the best technique is to lick from the bottom to the top, following the swirl of the candy.

No. 35 SEX & CANDY

INGREDIENTS
several heart-shaped lollipops

HERE'S HOW I THINK IT STARTED:

Caveman comes home, exhausted from another long day of hunting. The mastodon got away, and one of the other cavemen made fun of him—*"You throw spear like girl!"*—so he's a little cranky. He's wishing someone would hurry up and invent television. And beer. Cave romance is the last thing on his mind.

His cave spouse wants to show him the cool thing she gathered today with the other cave girls. It's a beehive, all nice and de-beed, and she's very excited about it, but she can tell he's just feigning interest to be polite. Suddenly, the hive breaks open. Honey spills out, making a mess all over the cave girl. At first they laugh about it, but then the cave guy gets an idea and starts to lick the honey off her skin.

And that was it. That was the invention of oral sex.

Honeylingus, in the old language.

That's my theory, anyway. I could be mistaken. However it started, though, sex has been sweeter ever since, don't you think?

Lucky for us, our forefathers also eventually created *candy*, and that's why we can now enjoy sugary treats without having to fight bees or get naked. But some inner part of us always remembers that amazing, delicious discovery by our ancient ancestors, and so those two concepts—sex and candy—are always locked together in our heads. I mean, really, when you see someone sucking on a lollipop, what do you think of? Let me rephrase that: *What does your guy think of* when he sees a stick of candy sliding in and out of your mouth?

You know the answer.

You can, if you wish, create this seduction with any kind of sweet you like, even something as messy as honey. But I recommend *lollipops* and specifically those cute heart-shaped suckers. So adorable! Buy a bag of them and, early in the week, start leaving a trail of lollipops around the house. One by one, your guy will find your sweet surprises in unlikely spots—in his favorite chair, under his pillow, tucked in a shoe—and every time, he'll smile and think of you.

So far, pure romance. But on Friday, plant a slightly more wicked idea in his head. Leave him a lolly with a note taped to it: *I'm going to teach you a whole new way to enjoy these things, tomorrow night at eight.*

Leave another note with a lollipop in his car Saturday morning. *Lick this! Practice for tonight.*

Suddenly, he's that cave guy again. He'll be running his Saturday errands with a silly grin on his face. Honey-lingus, indeed. He can't wait to get back to the cave with you.

Right after dinner, unwrap another lollipop and give it a long, lascivious lick. Lock eyes with him while you pop it in your mouth

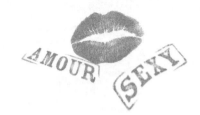
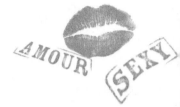
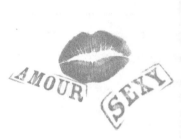
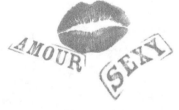

seduction no. 36

Panty Infractions

CULTURAL COCKTAIL: RUSSIA, FRANCE, ENGLAND

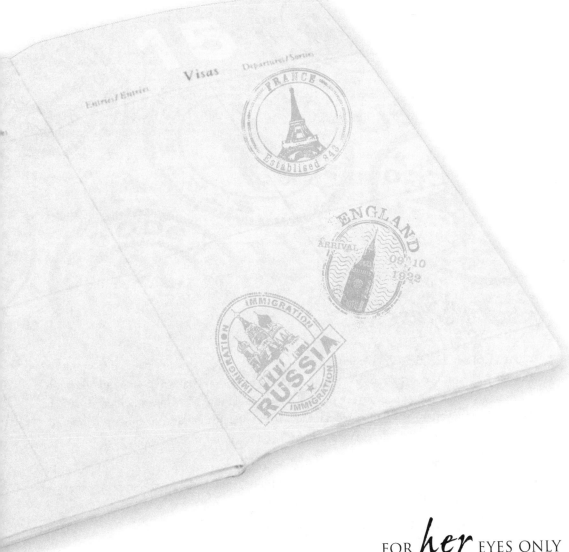

FOR *her* EYES ONLY

the hem. Jump and leap and make it clear that you know exactly what you're doing. Bend over to pick up a ball and then come up slowwwwly, back arched like a dancer. This kind of flirtation will work some powerful mojo on your guy, for two reasons. One, he can't touch you. (There's nothing like an obstacle, a net, for instance, to increase a man's desire for you.) Two, you're in a semipublic place, and that always makes men go wild, in a primal sort of way. When you're just a little bit bare like this, you're not just the sexiest thing in his life—you're the sexiest thing in the whole tribe. *And you're his.* Guys dig this. Makes them want to pound their chests.

So let your butt speak for itself. Let your cheeks peek out and tease your guy. Make him work up a sweat thinking about you. And then, when you climb back in the car, reach under your skirt and pull off your panties. Wrap them around a tennis ball and hand them to him. Giggle a little. Let him get a good, long look at you, then ask him to take you home.

And tell him he can skip the ice cream. Not the licking, just the ice cream.

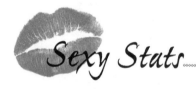

Sexy Stats

- Tatiana Golovin had the Wimbledon referee checking his rule book for "panty infractions" when she appeared on the court wearing red underwear. Wimbledon boasts a "predominantly white" dress code, though young players love to challenge it, including Ms. Golovin. She received the go-ahead to play after clearing her red panties with the referee in advance. Since the item in question is underwear, the referee ruled it didn't need to conform to the white rule.

- After the match, Tatiana fielded questions from reporters that inevitably began with, "Can I ask you about your knickers?" According to Tatiana, "They say red is the color that proves that you're strong and you're confident, so I'm happy with my red knickers."

- In tennis you "ace" your opponent by serving a ball he can't return.

- Tennis players may cause controversy with the color of their underwear, but the cut of their panties falls into four basic categories: low-rise, French cut, boy short, and tummy control.

- Female tennis players don't take their panties plain—the most popular tennis panty is called Fancy Pants.

No. 36 PANTY INFRACTIONS

INGREDIENTS
1 tennis outfit
1 pair sexy undies
1 tennis court
2 rackets
balls—plenty of balls

Do you want to know how to *REALLY* supercharge your sex life? Try writing books like this one. Seriously, my own relationship is never hotter than when I'm working on a new book. I spend months gathering erotic ideas and bedroom tips. I talk about sex with friends and experts. I'm always on the lookout for something that will inspire me and my readers. (And I have to test out these seductions, of course!)

I knew I had a winner the day I saw this headline: "Hotpants on parade as Wimbledon players sell tradition short." England's *Daily Mail* had an article on the top women players in the world's most prestigious tennis tournament, and it wasn't about how they played the game. It was about how they showed their booties! The short-shorts under their tennis skirts didn't break any regulations, strictly speaking, but *wow*—there was no way to miss the cheeks on display as these athletes flew around the grass. First, it was the little French girl, Tatiana Golovin, still a teenager when she created this fuss. The next day the Russians joined in, and the Americans.

Well, I hadn't been on a tennis court in more than ten years, but I knew I had to take this idea and run with it. The best seductions always start outside the bedroom, and they usually begin with something fun and flirtatious and completely surprising. Sure enough, this seduction knocked my guy off his feet—literally, he tripped and fell when he saw what I was up to—and it led to a memorable night of white-hot sex.

You might have to do what I did: that is, borrow some rackets and tennis whites from a friend who plays regularly. Talk your man into getting a little exercise this weekend. *"Hey, c'mon, it'll be fun! You know it'll be good for us, and you can buy me ice cream after."* Once you're on the court, the rest happens naturally as you run around chasing the ball. Just like Maria Sharapova and Serena Williams at Wimbledon, your skirt will start swaying and bouncing. And as your hemline swings, your sweetie will be unable to miss the luscious treat you've prepared for him. *It's your bum, mum.* Some of it, anyway. Exactly how much you display depends on your sense of modesty and degree of privacy. But at the very least—which is to say, the very *most*—you should be wearing some adorable sheer boy shorts. Not the big cotton kind. I mean something like Cosabella, or Victoria's Secret's amazing Cheekies, sexy boy short panties that reveal *just enough*, exposing about a quarter of your bottom. And that's if you're shy. To really whack your guy upside the head, there's no substitute for a thong.

Watch his eyes. You'll know when he's catching on. He'll do a double take, or miss a swing. (Or fall over, like my Jeff!) He'll gawk. And that's when you should really start to put on a show for him. Wink as you spin around, sending your skirt flying. Turn your back to him and flip up

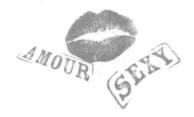
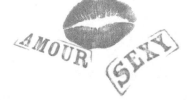
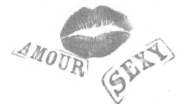
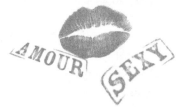
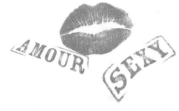
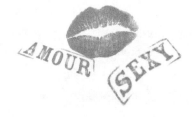
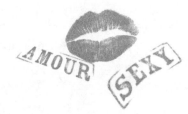

seduction no. 37

Skilled Hands

TROBRIAND ISLANDS, PAPUA NEW GUINEA

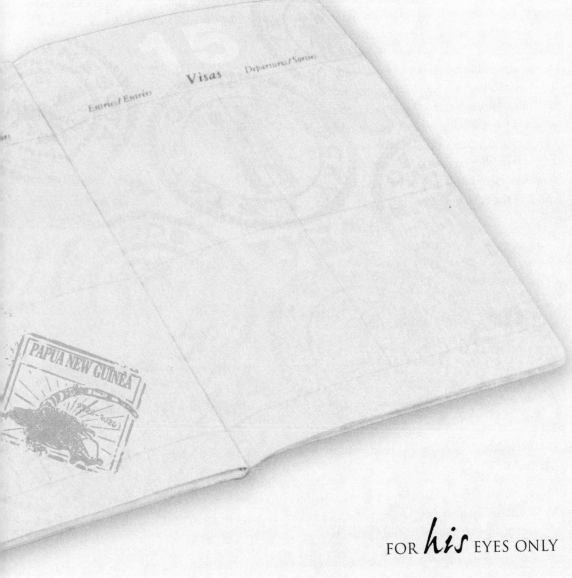

FOR *his* EYES ONLY

sensitivity of skin, because your palms are just close enough to generate a light charge of static electricity across the hairs on her arms. Slowly move your hands, hovering a few millimeters above her, generating warmth and a gentle tingle in her skin. This almost-a-tickle sensation will leave her itching for a scratch, and so you'll give her one. Nothing that will leave a welt, like the young Trobrianders do. Just drag your fingernails along her arms and down her back. In all the world, there are few things more satisfying than a good scratch massage. Gently scratch her scalp, shoulders, back, and legs. Reach between her thighs and lightly scratch her mound, while pressing the heel of your hand against her clit and lips. *Wow*, that's good, and it's guaranteed to get her hot. Finally, warm a little massage oil in your hands, then work it into the big muscles in her shoulders and neck. Squeeze the tension from her calves. And—most important of all—massage the ache out of her feet.

She's all yours now. She's warm, wet, wildly in love, and ready for you to take her island style. Roll her onto her back and lift her feet up over your shoulders. Make sure there's a pillow under her hips; a little extra elevation makes your job a lot easier. Slide inside her and rock your hips, back and forth, up and down, and don't rush the job. If you were living with the islanders, you'd know that there's no need for speed, because as long as you know how to say sweet words and deliver the occasional pretty present, there's always more sex to be had.

(Of course, if you really *were* living with the islanders, there's a good chance you two would be doing all this in front of an audience of other happy couples!)

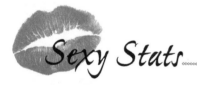

Sexy Stats

- Western massage therapists use scratching to "wake up" the skin after a particularly relaxing massage.

- "Scratching" is a technique used by hip-hop DJs who "scratch" the same note over and over on a record.

- As a boy reaches adolescence in the Trobriand Islands, he is given a gift of a penis gourd. Traditionally, men sheath their penises in hollowed-out, dried gourds tied to their bodies. The gourds are a symbol of hunting prowess.

- Scratching your lover can be slow and sensual, creating an intimate connection, or rougher and more primal, awakening the animal inside both of you.

- The average rainfall is 140 inches a year in the Trobriands. Rainy afternoons probably make for excellent courtship rituals.

№ 37 SKILLED HANDS

INGREDIENTS

love notes
1 blanket
candles (fireplace optional)

1 small flower (optional)
several pillows
massage oil

It's an exotic place where women rule. A place where youth and seduction and beauty are forms of wealth. It is, almost literally, the last place on Earth, at least according to Western history.

And it's where you're going to take your lover this week.

The Trobriand Islands are breathtakingly beautiful, if you don't mind a lot of tropical sweat with your white sand beaches. And here's the thing that really puts them on the cultural map: The islanders seem to be the least sexually inhibited people on the planet. They may not have much money, but there's plenty of sex to go around, assuming you bring the right gifts and say the right things. Lovemaking on Love Island requires a lot of sweet talk. And, interestingly, it almost always involves *scratching*.

Not just little scratches, either. They really dig in when they do the deed. If you're a young Trob, your buddies are going to check your back for marks and give you the island equivalent of the high five when they find them. It's proof of your prowess, you see, and if your girl actually drew blood, then *du-uu-ude*! You are the *Man*! And if you don't leave some passion marks on your girlfriend's back, then her friends are going to gossip about you, and not in a good way. How do you say *pansy* in Kilivila?

So you might be asking yourself right about now: Laura, are you expecting me to claw my sweetie like a horny alleycat? No. But in this week's seduction, you *are* going to use a special massage technique that involves scratching.

Start with a sweet written invitation early in the week. Leave it someplace she can't miss, like right next to her makeup mirror. *You're the love of my life!* it reads. *And I want to spend an evening alone with you—Saturday at 6.* Is anything blooming in your yard or neighborhood? Then pluck one single blossom, even something as simple as a dandelion, and put it on top of your note. The next day, leave another note, this time on her car seat: *I keep thinking about the time we met, and how you knocked me out when I first saw you. I love you.* Later in the week, send her an e-mail, or better, one of those online greeting cards, and tell her again, in just a few simple words, how beautiful she is.

When Saturday rolls around, set up a private *kwakwadu* for two. Throw a big blanket and some pillows on the living room floor. Put on soft lights and soft music. Light some candles, or if you have a fireplace, spark it up. Try to re-create the crazy make-out sessions you two had when you first fell in love. Kiss her and tell her how important she is to you. Tell her you love her. And after a while, tell her you want to try a new massage you read about. Make sure she's comfortable on the pillows and that the room is warm enough for bare skin.

Start by placing your hands over her arm but *not quite touching her*. This technique heightens the

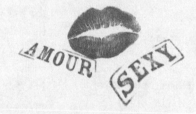
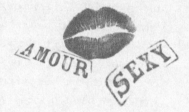

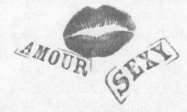
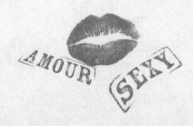
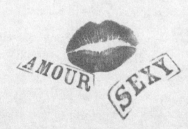

seduction no. 38

MySexySpace

EUROPE

FOR *her* EYES ONLY

$

Start in your bathroom. Lots of light there, right? Practice posing and shooting. Get a feel for working with mirrors, the big one over the sink, the portable full-length mirror, even your makeup mirror. Shoot your back and your bare bottom. Remember, no picture will escape from the camera unless you like it, so experiment! Nipples out or covered by one arm? Face serious or smiling? It's amazing what a simple change in posture can do to breasts. Reach up, lean back, bend over, and watch how they change.

Arrange for some private time in the house and move your mirror to the bedroom. Play dress-up: jeans, dresses, heels, lingerie. When you like what you see in the mirror, aim your camera at it and squeeze. Move the mirror around the house, looking for the perfect spot to pose: a place where the light is bright enough to turn the flash off, but soft, flooding through sheer curtains or bouncing off walls, creating gentle shadows along the curves of your body. Have a glass of wine, maybe, and imagine your guy looking at you through the lens.

Do you have some outdoor privacy? Then move your mirror outside. Shirt open, *click*. Panties and bra, *click*. Jump off a chair and catch yourself midleap, *click*. Wrap the garden hose around you like a snake; turn it on and spray yourself, laughing madly, *click*. Pose on a lounge chair, soaking wet and as naked as you dare, *click*.

The secret to taking great pictures is to take a lot of pictures and keep only one out of ten. Don't aim for perfection. And don't worry about being sexy; the sexiness is already there, inside you. Just keep the ones you like best, the shots where you look happy and comfortable. Print one of them and leave it on your guy's pillow just before bed Wednesday night. Print another one and sneak it to him after Thursday's dinner. Print another and hand it to him Friday morning. *Wow.* You'll see a big difference in his behavior right away. That's because he suddenly can't stop thinking of you. He can't help but notice how attractive you are. And the boldness, the sheer self-confidence your pictures display, well, that's a crazy turn-on for any man. Just wait until he sees your whole collection Saturday night, scrolling by in a slide show on your monitor, or printed and taped to the bedroom walls.

I have a feeling things are really going to . . . *click*.

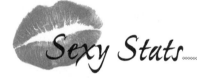

Sexy Stats

- For inspiration, check out www.IShotMySelf.com, a public art apparatus that features hundreds of thousands of erotic self-portraits.

- Boudoir is a term used to describe a revealing style of photography. Implied nudity is common, as is the subject showing part of their undergarments while still dressed.

- The French pioneered erotic photography, producing nude postcards that became the subject of an officer's letter to President Abraham Lincoln after they were found in the possession of United States troops, according to *An Underground Education* by Richard Zacks.

- A self-portrait is a representation of an artist, drawn, painted, photographed, or sculpted by the artist. The medium became popular during the early Renaissance in the mid-1400s. Better and cheaper mirrors became available, and many painters, sculptors and printmakers tried some form of self-portraiture.

No. 38 MYSEXYSPACE

INGREDIENTS
1 digital camera
1 portable full-length mirror
tripod and remote control (optional)

Out of all the seductions in the book, this one just might be the most fun. (For the *seducer*, I mean! Because for the seducee, naturally, they are *all* fun.)

You get to be creative and artistic and sexy. You get to be fabulous. You get to be *that girl*—the hot one, the cute one, the one in the ads, the one the camera loves. This week, you get to direct your own photo shoot.

Every day, all over the world, people stick their arms out as far as they can, turn the camera back on themselves, and click. Smiling tourists, drunk girlfriends, happy partiers are posted by the gazillions on the Internet. What these self-portraits lack in technical perfection is made up in pure joy. There is life in these pictures. People love them, and here's why: *because the subjects are in control.* When you take your own picture, you get to decide when to snap the shutter. There's none of that forced-smile eyelid-fluttering waiting-for-the-damned-flash anxiety that makes so many group shots look phony. No bad angles or goofy hair—at least not for long, because bad shots get erased in an instant. In the end, all you have left is photos where *you think you look good.* You decide which pictures make you happy and throw away the rest.

That's the secret behind the gift you're making for your guy this week. He already loves the average everyday you, so he is going to just flip for pictures of the very best, happiest you. Especially when you're, um, not exactly fully dressed.

I was inspired to try this by a famous Paris-based photographer named Uwe Ommer. A few years ago, he started letting his subjects use his gear to take pictures of themselves. The results were wildly sexy, for all the reasons I mentioned above. These girls—not all of them professional models—got to take the pictures at the moment they thought they looked their best. And you can see that glorious sense of satisfaction all over their faces. They're not the least bit self-conscious, even when nearly nude, because they didn't take the picture until they felt like they looked good. Exuberance and spontaneity make these pictures hot in a very modern way, like a mash up of Facebook and *Playboy.*

You'll need a digital camera, of course. You can make this whole seduction work by shooting handheld with a bargain camera, or even a cell phone camera. But if you really want to explore your creativity, there are two accessories you might want to buy or borrow: a small tripod, to hold the camera still and a remote control, to make it click at a distance. And there's one more critical ingredient. If you're going to be *that girl*, you can't be shooting from the end of your extended arm. You need to see yourself. You need to know the moment when you look your hottest. And that means you will be taking most of these pictures while posing in front of a mirror. I found a full-length, over-the-door mirror for less than $20, and it weighs so little that I can carry it all over the house.

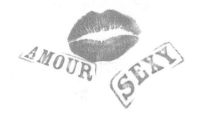
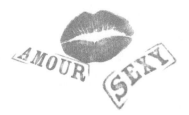
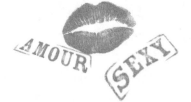
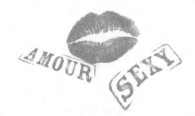

seduction no. *39*

Splish, Splosh

CULTURAL COCKTAIL: NEW YORK, UNITED KINGDOM

FOR *her* EYES ONLY

that get there? Dip your finger in and suck it clean. *"Yummy, so sweet . . ."* Dip in again with two fingers and hold them in front of him. When he moves in to take it, pull back and smear it onto your breast. As he leans forward to lick you clean, take another scoop and smoosh it into the back of his neck as you pull him toward you.

Offer the container to him and start sploshing: *cover* yourselves in pudding. Throw a glob at his chest and use your breasts to rub it in. Give him a pudding face paint à la *Braveheart*. Laugh at how silly you both look. Play!

Set a towel on the edge of the tub and tell him to sit on it and you sit between his feet. Take a handful of pudding and smear it up and down his shaft. If he wasn't hard already, he will be as soon as your lips and tongue go to work licking and sucking along his length.

Look up at him and smile, tell him how turned on this gets you and how good he tastes. Swirl your tongue around the underside of his erection as you suck; you don't want to miss a single drop.

When your mouth is full of, um, pudding, show him your tongue, then *slowly tilt your head back and swallow.*

When the pudding's gone, or you're both so worked up you can't wait any longer, turn on the shower. You'll have pudding in your hair, your nose—everywhere—but try to keep it out of your vagina. Sugar can be a big no-no in the *vajay-jay.*

Once you're squeaky clean, jelly bean, towel off and take things up in the bedroom, you've got some serious calories to burn off, and a game of *Hide the Salami* is the perfect workout.

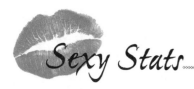

Sexy Stats

- Vanilla is the number one selling fragrance in women's cosmetics, and there's a reason. The sex researcher, Havelock Ellis, discovered that the scent of vanilla increases blood flow to the penis by 8 percent when he noticed vanilla pod factory workers who were in a constant state of arousal. No wonder turnover is so low at those places.

- Kim Basinger and Mickey Rourke serve up some hot sploshing action in the movie *9 1/2 Weeks*. On the floor. In front of the refrigerator. Honey, anyone?

- Wet and messy fetish (WAM) is a form of sexual fetishism whereby a person becomes aroused when substances are deliberately and generously applied to the naked skin, or to the clothes people are wearing.

No. 39 SPLISH, SPLOSH

INGREDIENTS

1 large bowl of vanilla pudding
candles
towels

1 bathtub
1 large basket or bowl
sparkling cider or champagne

IF YOU MAKE A MESS, YOU HAVE TO CLEAN IT UP.

That's what our parents always said. Only thing is, ladies, this time you're going to *want* to clean up your mess. Because it's going to be all over your man. Don't worry, though, he'll happily return the favor.

Have you ever heard something so kinky and unbelievable that your first reaction is, "No freaking way, that is not for me!"? That was my reaction when I first read an article about sploshing.

Why should you be interested in some crazy kink popularized by people who call sausages "bangers"? Why would you want to try something that's going to make a sticky mess in your house? For the same reason I did: *curiosity*. It sounded so crazy I *had* to try it.

First of all, I loved the word. Just say it: *sploshing*. It sounds like what it is—smearing something messy on your naked skin and squishing around with your partner. Sploshers use anything from milk to honey to spaghetti and meatballs. Stay with me, ladies, because once you get past the "we don't play with our food" mentality, sploshing can be fun and silly, pretty darn delicious, and sexy.

Here's what you do.

Buy a tub of vanilla pudding and a bottle of sparkling cider or champagne. Make sure your bathtub is clean and set your candles around the bathroom. Go a little crazy with the candles— a bag of one hundred tea lights costs a couple of bucks—put a few in the sink, several along the counter and along the back of the toilet. Shut off the AC and turn on a space heater if it's chilly.

Place a bowl of pudding next to the tub and drape a towel over it to hide it. Make it pretty, like you've got a relaxing bath planned for the two of you.

Set the champagne bottle and glasses on the counter and go fetch your guy. Take him by the hand and say, *"Baby, you look exhausted. I've got just the thing to perk you up."* Lead him into the candlelit bathroom and let his eyes adjust to the darkness. *How romantic*, he thinks, *I'm the luckiest guy in the world.* Ask him to open the bottle. Make him feel useful, and let him appreciate his lady being in charge.

Turn off the water when the tub is about two inches full. Tell him you'd like to propose a toast, *"To fun and games."*

Clink.

Undress and invite him to join you in the bathtub. You're naked, and after that toast you just made sure he'll pretty much do whatever you say. Sit in the warm bit of water and make room for him to sit facing you. Wrap your arms and legs around his naked body and squeeze.

Kiss his neck, *"Mmmm, you're salty . . ."* Reach down and pull out the pudding. Now, how did

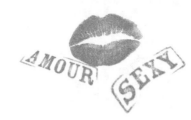

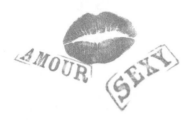

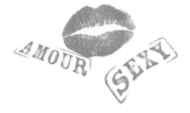

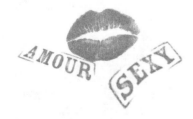

seduction no. 40

Rhythm King

CARIBBEAN

FOR *his* EYES ONLY

offbeat. It forces you to walk just a little slower than is natural for you. It throws you off. To compensate, your hips have to swing out farther. Your whole body sways. Before you know it, you're dancing with your sweetie. Crush up against her, pelvis to pelvis, Jamaican style. Slowly turn and crouch down, so that your butt is grinding on her. All you need is some dreads and a tan, and you'd be a Caribbean rent-a-gent already.

Toss your boopsie onto the sheets and make a big show of stacking two pillows on the edge of the bed. Grab her legs and pull her to you. Lift her hips like a manly man and then drop them right on the pile of pillows, with her legs up, feet over your shoulders. Mmm—that lovely *punaana* is now exposed and elevated right before you. Get on your knees and show her what you can do with your tongue. Eat her like you're starving; make her feel your hunger. Go ahead and play with yourself while you're dining. Make yourself hard. Because in ten minutes, you have to be ready to stand up and deliver. And ten minutes after that, you're going to drop down and lick

again. And ten minutes after *that* . . . well, just stick to the Ten-Minute Rule. The professional lovers of the islands keep switching it up, never running any game more than ten minutes. The ladies approve.

The ladies also dig the round-and-round hip action of their island lovers. It's not about pumping in and out. The beachboys follow the slow thump of the music they love, gliding their hips on the offbeat, side to side, up and down. Your erection should roll in a circle around the outside edge of the vagina, like you're stirring a pot with a really thick-handled spoon. It works so well because that's where the nerves are, concentrated in the lips and outer couple of inches of the *pum-pum*.

Size doan matta when you got de skill, mon. And with the grindsman skills you've just shown her—every weekend is going to be a Caribbean vacation.

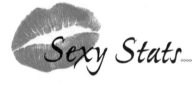 *Sexy Stats*

- Jamaica's Hedonism I and Hedonism II resorts (there is a III under construction) are clothing-optional, adults-only playgrounds. Couples report that a sexually uninhibited vacation at Hedo is just what they needed to rev things up back in the real world.

- In Jamaica, if you perform oral sex on a woman, you are *bowing* to her. And if you're really good at it, you'll bring her to *agony, mon.*

- Make circles: Men who thrust in a circular motion—rather than straight in and out—have greater ejaculatory control.

- Casanova knew that a rocking motion was the way to send a woman straight to ecstasy.

- Going down on a woman isn't a race; most like it slow, especially at first. Flatten your tongue, use plenty of saliva, and slowly lick everywhere but the clit. She'll let you know when you've found a good spot and when you can speed up.

No. **40** RHYTHM KING

INGREDIENTS
2 or more reggae songs
2 pillows
2 loose hips

THERE ARE A LOT OF THINGS THAT MAKE A man into a magnificent lover. Though it might surprise you to know what's *not* at the top of the list: a big penis.

For most women, I'll bet that's not even in the top ten. Seriously. But if there is any truly essential ingredient, it's *confidence*. To be a great lover, you have to believe you're a great lover. Maybe that explains why women have been flocking to the Caribbean for wild vacations, heading home thrilled, throbbing, utterly exhausted—and eager for a repeat visit.

The beachboys of Jamaica and the Dominican Republic think they're the best lovers in the world. Just ask them! *Hey, evahbody know it, mon; did you no' see* How Stella Got Her Groove Back?

But confidence isn't everything. Those Caribbean Kings have a few sexy secrets that make women melt, and you're going to use them all week long. It all starts with *de riddum*, that offbeat rhythm of reggae music you hear from shore to shore in the Antilles. Reggae is sex music, pure and simple. Dancing to it is really just a vertical interpretation of the horizontal boogie, set to a relaxed tempo. It's not easy for a guy to pace himself during sex, when every instinct is telling you to push push push. But reggae's sharp offbeat accents and missing one-beat are contrary to most modern music, so it throws you, just a little. The harmonic simplicity and repetitious chords make it hypnotic. It all forces you to *slow down* to a pace that is exactly right for a woman's pleasure.

Oh, yeah, you are definitely going to need a couple of reggae songs. Look for Maxi Priest or anything by Bob Marley.

Here's another secret of the Caribbean: *praise*. Lots of it. The boys flirt shamelessly, piling one compliment on top of another. It's outrageous, unbelievable . . . and delicious. Women love to hear it, even when they know it's an exaggeration. So start your seduction early in the week with a sweet, slightly over-the-top love note: *You are the best thing that ever happened to me, and I'm sorry if I forget to say it often enough.* Leave it where your lady will find it, taped to the ice cream or slipped into her purse. The next day, send her an e-mail: *I can never get enough of you. I love you.* Try this in a text message: *You turn me on.*

Wow! In Kingston, she'd say, "*Wa mek yu sweet so?*" How come you're so sweet?

Keep up the love talk all week. It's easy. Just think about all the things that first knocked you out when you met her and tell her about them. Don't be shy, and do it in plain English; if you thought she had an ass to die for, say so. Tell her how much you love her kisses, her hair, the way her nipples sometimes pop under a tight shirt. Even the most refined woman likes to know she still inspires a boner, *brudda*. As the weekend approaches, ask her out, and make it clear that you have every intention of getting her naked and on her back.

When the time comes, pipe a hot *ragga* through your stereo. Don't just listen. *Feel it.* Step to the

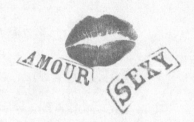
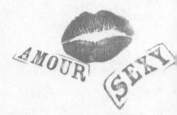

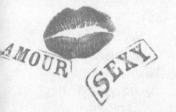
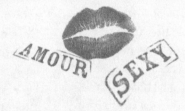

seduction no. **41**

Brush Strokes

CHINA

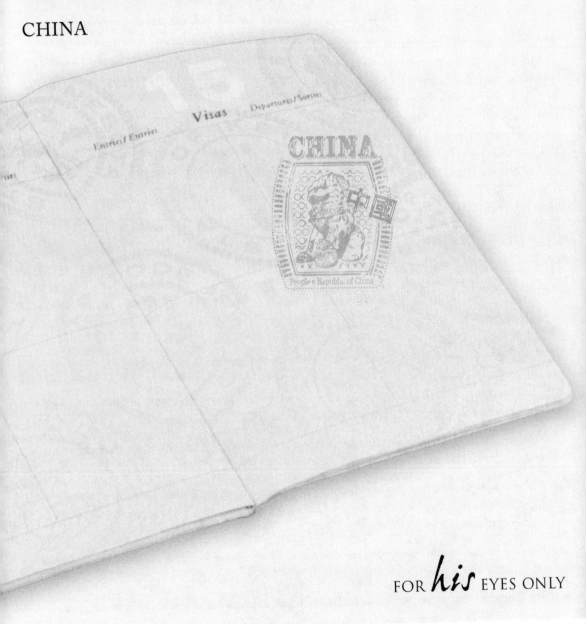

FOR *his* EYES ONLY

$

paintbrush in water and draw a symbol across her chest. When she asks what you've drawn, tell her it's the symbol for *Sexy*. Dip the brush in water once more and swirl it around her nipples . . . first one, then the other. Tell her that was the symbol for *Luscious*. Part her robe and run your wet paintbrush over her tummy. *"That's the symbol for desire,"* you tell her, letting the brush rest just above her mound.

By now, your girl will be squirming in her chair. Dip the brush in water again and tell her to spread her thighs . . . then run the brush over her clit. Tease her with the paintbrush, making gentle brushstrokes over her lower lips before returning to her clit. Go over her clit again and again, dipping the brush in water between strokes. The water and her own arousal will soon have her eager for the art lesson to end and the lovemaking to begin.

When she can't take the teasing anymore, tell her you have a different kind of brush to use on her. Get undressed . . . slowly. . . . When you are naked, dip your fingers in the and rub water over your penis. Then grab the chair and pull her toward you. Press the tip of your erection against her wetness and then brush it against her clit, using all of that moisture to "paint" her the way you did with the paintbrush. When she is eagerly tilting her hips up to meet those gentle strokes, put your hands under her bottom and slide *against* her, but not *inside* her. Not yet. Keep your strokes gentle and slow until neither of you can stand it anymore and she is rocking against you and whimpering with need. Then whisper those words that will satisfy her heart's greatest desire: *"I want to be inside you."*

Now that's what it means to be truly enlightened.

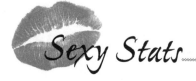

Sexy Stats

- The oldest sex manuals in the world are the *Handbooks of Sex* written more than five thousand years ago by the legendary Chinese emperor Huang-Ti.

- Ancient Chinese taoist lovemaking practices were based on the harmony of yin (female essence) and yang (male essence).

- Chinese women are often considered demure and submissive, but China has many sensual legends involving strong warrior women. One such woman was Hua Mu Lan, who found love on the battlefield.

- Chinese erotica can be traced back to depictions of lovemaking found on sculpted bricks from around A.D. 100.

- The Chinese word for sensual pleasure, including all the varieties of sex, is *shufu*, which means physical well-being or comfort.

No. 41 BRUSH STROKES

INGREDIENTS
1 Zen Board (also called a Buddha Board)
1 chair
towel

1 paintbrush
1 small bowl of water
candles

IF YOU THINK OF TRANQUILLITY AND
meditation when you think of Zen, think again!
The sensual secrets of the Far East are connected
to that higher plane of self-awareness known
as Zen. Being self-aware means living in the
moment in order to achieve your heart's greatest
desires. Since there is nothing a woman loves
more than being surprised with a thoughtful
gift, you will need to make a trip to your local
art supply store or website for a Zen Board. For
less than the cost of two tickets to a martial arts
movie, you are going to satisfy your lady's desires
and create a memorable night of *wild* passion for
both of you. Who knew Zen could be so sexy?

It's no secret that women love to be seduced
with words—there is something wickedly
arousing about exploring your passion through
communication. But rather than *telling* her what
you're going to do, you are going to *paint* it! Zen
Boards are a different kind of canvas—you use
water instead of paint. The image appears as black
against the white paper but, within a couple of
minutes, the picture evaporates. Zen is all about
letting go . . . so whatever you paint disappears
before your eyes, leaving only a memory behind.
You're going to create a sensual memory that will
linger long after the water has evaporated!

Tell your girl you would like to make a date with
her for a special "art class." In the week leading up
to the big event, leave her a couple of notes on the
refrigerator or tucked into her purse to remind
her of your plans. *I can't wait to study your form.*

Or, *Will you pose naked for me?* She will be amused
by your playful words, but she will never be able
to anticipate what you have in store for her.

On the day of your date, ask her to slip into a
robe or a shirt that buttons up the front. Prepare
the bedroom with a kitchen chair near the bed
and a small bowl of water within arm's reach.
Lay a towel on the chair, put on some soft music,
and light a few candles around the room. Place
the Zen Board and paintbrush on the chair and
then invite your girl into your "art studio." She
will be intrigued, wondering what in the world
you have in mind. Have her sit in the chair as
you sit across from her on the bed and explain
how the Zen Board works.

Your Zen Board will come with a booklet of
Chinese-Japanese *kanji* symbols that represent
words. As your girl practices on the Zen Board,
you can show her various symbols to paint.
Choose symbols for words that reflect how
you feel about her, such as *Love, Happiness*, and
Beauty. Have her draw the symbol on the Zen
Board *before* you tell her what it means. She will
be mesmerized as the water evaporates from the
board, and all of the day's stresses will begin to
melt away. This is Zen . . . this is living in the
moment.

After a few minutes, tell her you want to draw
some symbols, too. *This is where you get to have
some fun!* Take the Zen Board and paintbrush
from her and lay the board aside. Slowly open
her robe so that her breasts are exposed. Dip the

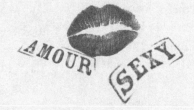
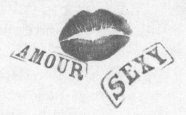

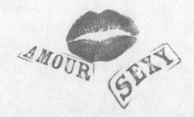

seduction no. 42

Double Exposure

MIAMI, FLORIDA, USA

FOR *her* EYES ONLY

He could escape, of course. But he won't. He wants to see where this is going. More than that, he wants to surrender to you. And he won't be sorry he did.

Kneel on the pillow in front of him. Drag your fingernails across the front of his boxers. Feel his package stirring underneath the fabric. Give him a gentle squeeze. Now press your cheek up against the beast hiding inside and slowly slide your face from side to side. *Ahhh*. He's breathing harder now. His penis is growing, pressing against the cloth, and when you take the tip of it and place it between your teeth, still wrapped in fabric, you'll feel it twitch. Pull down his underwear, an inch at a time, and once his erection is free, slide it into your mouth and work it, in and out, wet and hard. Take your time.

Stand up and turn around. Tease him with your bottom. Rub it against his crotch and then step away. Do it a few times. Make him tug on the ropes and shove his hips forward, as he tries to get his arrow closer to the target. It's okay to giggle when you dodge his thrusts.

Finally, free his wrists and bring him to the centerpiece of your seduction. It's a big mirror, leaning up against a wall or dresser. Put the pillow in front of it and get down on all fours, with your face near the glass. Tell him to get behind you, and "*Put it in me, right now. I need it in me hard.*"

And that's when he figures it out. The mirror has magic. He can have sex with you, and *he can watch himself having sex with you*. He's just inches away from it, too. It's almost like having sex with another couple, close enough to touch. In fact, you're so close to the mirror you could almost start making out with that other beautiful girl in the room. He loves you, and only you, but for a brief while, he gets to share you with that other guy.

He's gone through the looking glass. But this sure isn't Wonderland. It's *wonder-when-we-can-do-this-again* land.

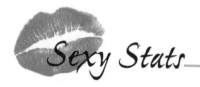

Sexy Stats

- From the sexy heat of South Beach to the hot Latino beats in the nightclubs, Miami's combination of cultures makes it the sexiest city in the United States, according to MSN Travel.

No. 42 DOUBLE EXPOSURE

INGREDIENTS

1 large mirror
1 large throw pillow
1 soft rope, 4 feet long
  (optional: scarves, neckties, panty hose)

2 kitchen chairs
candles
1 pair boxers

A FRIEND OF MINE CALLED ME FROM MIAMI, where she was on vacation. She was trying to keep her voice low, but she could barely contain her excitement. "It was him, I know it was," she whispered. Her date had wangled an invitation to one of Miami's notorious sex clubs, and she had seen a Very Important Person, a nationally known politician. *And he was wearing leather chaps.* Ugh. There are very few people, we decided, who truly look good in assless pants. This guy was definitely not one of them.

But I was much more interested in hearing about what goes on inside one of those clubs. You can find them anywhere powerful and rich people congregate, high-end places where members, almost always couples, let go of their inhibitions and get kinky in public. The appeal is not obvious to everyone.

In case you're starting to get a little antsy right now, let me put your mind at ease. I am not going to suggest you take your sweetie to a swingers' club this week!

But here's the thing that draws some folks to places like that Miami club. First, the act of sexual surrender—giving complete control of your sexual pleasure to someone else—can be awesome. And second, it's just mind-blowing to *watch sex happen.* You're going to make both of those things come true for your partner this week.

Stop by the hardware store and get a short length of soft nylon rope. One day this week, hand your guy a knife and ask for his help cutting the rope in two. When he asks what it's for, look him in the eye and tell him the truth. *"Oh, honey, I'm going to tie you up with it this weekend!"* Smile, kiss him on the cheek, and walk away, leaving him to ponder just how much you were kidding. (The correct answer is not at all.)

Saturday night, tell him you have a few surprises for him, starting with a bath. Once he's in the tub, start setting up the scene of your seduction. When everything's in place, put a large pillow next to the tub. On it is a pair of boxer shorts, the two sections of rope, and a note that says, *Put on the boxers and bring the rest to the bedroom.* Wow. Gulp! Now he's *really* starting to wonder how much you were kidding. (The answer is still the same.)

When he walks into the bedroom, he'll see a sight that is at once stunning and slightly confusing. Two kitchen chairs sit in the middle of the floor, back to back, about three feet apart. Candlelight flickers on your skin, and there is a *lot* of skin exposed, set off by black lingerie. Tell your man to hand you the ropes and then drop the pillow at your feet. Make him stand between the chairs. Take one rope and loop it around his wrist, then through the opening on the back of one chair. Tie a knot. Repeat with his other wrist.

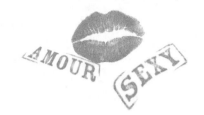
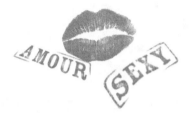

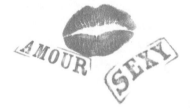

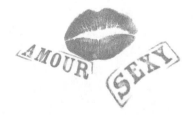
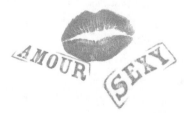

seduction no. 43

Two Nips Up

GREAT BRITAIN

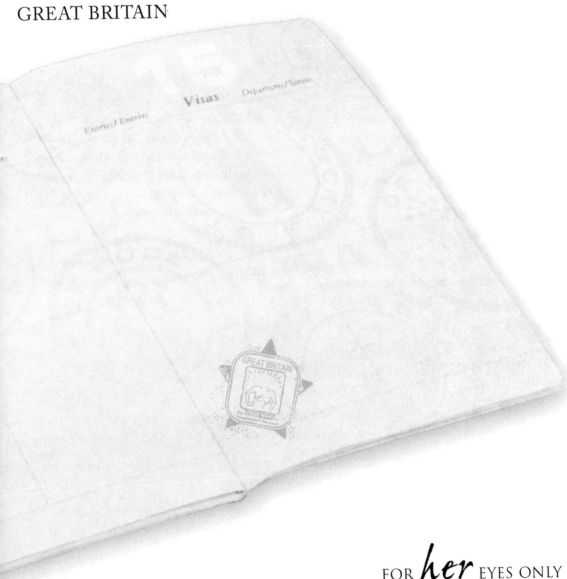

FOR *her* EYES ONLY

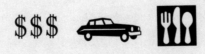

white blouse, extra unbuttoned. And under *that*—nothing but pretty temporary tats or stick-on jewels around your nipples. Just before you go into the restaurant, flash him and smile. Will you flash him again at the table? (Will you maybe even let the cute waiter catch a glimpse?) There is more to the evening than peekaboo. Let your guy know he can expect a special treat later. If he minds his manners.

When you get home and get undressed, push him back on the bed, straddle his hips, and show him Betty's Bells, the two small cups connected by a light chain. Apply a few drops of lubricant to the edges of the cups, press them to your breasts, and squeeze to force the air out. Watch his eyes pop as your nipples start to swell. Watch his jaw drop as you lift the lube over your head and pour it, dramatically and excessively, over your breasts. Feel him getting hard underneath you as you rub the lube all over your chest.

Hang your breasts over his face and shake them. Tug on the chain hanging between them—*what a feeling!*—and encourage him to do the same. For him, it's an incredible visual feast, but for you it's something more, something that combines tickling and pulling with an intense sensation of suckling, something that focuses your mind onto your buzzing nipples.

Slowly scoot down his legs so that the chain drags across his chest and stomach. Slide it up and around his erect penis. Press your breasts and your aching nips against his shaft. If you dare, loop the chain under his testicles and lift, ever so gently, creating some erotic tension between your most tender parts and his.

There is a limit to how long you can wear your new toys, and that limit is different for each woman. When they come off, your man will be knocked out by their size. They're swollen, bigger than ever, almost a caricature of an aroused aureole. (It's temporary. Unless you start making a serious habit of it.) *You* will be astonished by their extreme sensitivity, also temporary.

And both of you will have rediscovered your affection for those magnificent, sensual, lovely, and praiseworthy breasts.

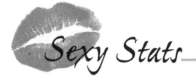

Sexy Stats

- London isn't in a fog when it comes to the availability of sex products. The most popular items for breast dress-up are nipple dust, false nipples, diamond nipple tassels, and cleavage enhancers.

- According to a recent survey by the bra maker Triumph, 57 percent of Englishwomen need a D-cup or larger, giving them the biggest breasts in Europe.

- Make your hot spots blush with Benefit's Benetint, created in 1977 when an exotic dancer requested a long-lasting product to stain her nipples pink during her performance.

- The Page 3 of the British newspaper the *Sun* features photographs of a topless female model on the third page of the newspaper. When the Page 3 girl went topless on November 17, 1970, sales rose 40 percent to 2.1 million copies within a year.

- B.S.H stands for *British standard handful*, a unit used to measure mammary glands and is often uttered when a gentleman is impressed by their size. *My word, that lady has large breasts. I say, she certainly has a B.S.H.*

INGREDIENTS

1 eye-catching bra
1 jacket
nipple clamps or 2 nipple sucklers
(like Betty's Bells, from
www.a-womans-touch.com)

1 sheer white shirt
2 temporary nipple tattoos, or "tittytats"
1 bottle of adult lubricant, like Wet or Astroglide

A COUPLE OF YEARS AGO, JEFF AND I TOOK a vacation—excuse me, we went on holiday—in London. Less than two days into the trip, we found ourselves in a pub, when Jeff turned to me with a perfectly straight face and asked, *"What is up with all the cleavage in this town?"*

I burst out laughing, because I had been thinking the same thing myself. England, it seems, is the Land o' Bosoms.

They were everywhere. And not in that barely-covered, popping-out style you sometimes see in Miami or LA. What we were seeing was lots of *décolletage*—otherwise demure dresses and suits cut deep in front to show the delicious curve of the female breast. Big, small, and in between, British lasses are happy to open an extra button to show their bits. The lads, it should be noted, are delighted with this arrangement.

This week, you and your man are going to celebrate your breasts. To get the "t" party started, you will need a beautiful new bra and some, uh, accessories. What kind of accessories? Well, I'm going to use two words that sound much scarier than they really are: *nipple clamps*.

I know what you're thinking. *Ouch!* But all your fears and concerns will be dispelled once you see the latest in breast fashions. Temporary nipple tattoos. Jeweled appliqués. Chocolate pasties with peanut butter adhesive. Yum. And yes, traditional nipple clamps, padded, spring-loaded, and adjustable. Consider purchasing Betty's

Bells. These are small cups made of clear plastic, about the size of shot glasses. They fit over your nipples, and stay attached through gentle vacuum pressure. More comfortable than metal clamps, they also create an extraordinary visual effect guaranteed to mesmerize your guy: *Your nipples get drawn into the cups.* The slight vacuum causes your nipples to extend and swell, which looks awesome and makes them astonishingly sensitive.

Of course, choosing a sex toy is a highly personal decision, and you should pick whatever appeals to you. From here on, wherever you read "Betty's Bells," imagine your own favorite breast toy.

Begin your week of breast worship by putting the girls on display. Make sure your guy sees a lot of them around the house this week, in revealing tops, lingerie, packed into brassieres, or set free. You might think they're past their prime, maybe too petite, but your guy *adores* them. He is grateful to have them around, and he'll love it every time you casually stroll past him with your shirt off or open. To call attention to them, stand in front of the mirror one morning, just before he leaves for work, and tweak your nipples, right in front of him. *"Wow, these seem extrasensitive today,"* you tell him. *"Do they seem different to you, honey?"* Your man will spend the rest of the day with exactly one thought careening around his noggin: *Extra Sensitive Nipples.* Hah! It will be a wonder if he can get any work done.

Go out to dinner Saturday night and wear an outfit with a jacket. Under that, your sheerest

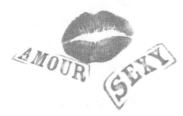

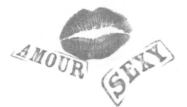

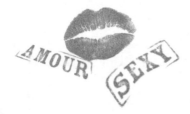

seduction no. **44**

Dining in the Dark

SWITZERLAND, GERMANY

FOR *his* EYES ONLY

$

some music. Bring your sweetie to the dining table and then invite her to *put on a sleep mask*. You've put her curiosity into overdrive now. She's blindfolded and wearing her ultracomfy T-shirt, with a big napkin or two covering her bare thighs. She can hear you setting plates on the table, and she can smell something delicious. *Don't tell her what's on the menu.* Just explain the relative position of everything: meat at three o'clock, vegetable at nine o'clock, water glass at one o'clock, et cetera. Let her feel your face to prove that you, too, now have a mask over your eyes. Kiss her. And start to eat.

In the beginning, it will be pure hilarity. Some things will go splat. Soon, though, you'll learn to feed yourselves, and that's when it's time to start trying to feed each other. As you work it out, you'll find that there's more to this sensuous experience than delicious tastes and surprising textures. You're also touching her face and caressing her lips. You're sucking yummy drips off her fingers. You're experiencing your sweetie with a new perspective, just like you did with the food, and she is feeling you in a whole new way. Like I said, it's *sexy*.

Get up and dance. Slowly lead her to the sofa. Of course, in anticipation of this date you've already cleared the room of any shin-banging objects and tossed a blanket over the couch. Dessert is already waiting on an end table. I recommend *cheesecake*. Not only one of the most delicious things ever invented by man, but also the perfect consistency for macking in the dark—soft, slightly sticky, won't dribble.

The masks can come off now. Lights should be off, too. Use your tongue to explore for dropped bits. *Oh, there must be some cheesecake down here, right on your panties, why don't I take a look and . . . mmm, yum, what's this?*

Take a nibble. Give a lick. Show her how educated your tongue has become in just the last hour. Offer her a taste of your own personal specialty, the famous *bony cannelloni*, with the creamy surprise in the center. Use your newly enhanced senses to explore her skin, her breasts, her clit. You promised to take care of everything tonight, and a meal like this isn't complete without a breath-sucking, toe-curling, thigh-trembling orgasm.

So rare. Yet so well done.

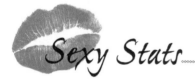

Sexy Stats

- The original lights-out restaurant is called Blinde Kuh, which is German for the game Blind Man's Buff, and most of the restaurant staff are visually impaired.

- Sausages are the most popular German food to eat in the dark. Not surprising, since there are more than fifteen hundred different varieties of sausage across Germany. Which leads me to wonder, what other "sausages" are being sampled in complete darkness?

- Dark dining is sweeping the globe. Young professionals in the UK, France, and Australia are meeting potential partners, very literally, for blind dates.

- When you dine in the dark, you talk more softly, listen more closely, and touch more gently. With the flick of a switch, you feel and act sexier.

INGREDIENTS
2 large cloth napkins
2 great take-out dinners, with dessert
2 sleep masks or blindfolds

I ADMIT IT. I THOUGHT THIS WAS *CRAZY* THE first time I heard about it. Eating in a pitch-dark restaurant? Sounds, I don't know, messy and dangerous. (Of course, my impression may have been colored by the fact that I first saw this done on a TV crime show, in which one of the diners is murdered at the table in the darkness and— you can guess what's next—can't you?—*nobody saw a thing.* Cue the scary music!)

In real life, it turns out that dining in the dark is *fun.* It's one of the few surefire ways to gain a whole new perspective on something you think you know well. Food is our first sensual pleasure; you've been indulging in it your entire life. But when you can't see it, a meal takes on several new dimensions. You have to concentrate on how food feels and how it smells. You become much more aware of texture and temperature and aftertaste. And, of course, you first have to get it into your mouth, an experience that can quickly turn dinner into comedy.

The first lights-out restaurant was launched in Zurich, Switzerland, at the turn of the millennium, and the phenomenon quickly spread to Germany. Adventurous eaters loved the opportunity to try something new and expand their senses. It didn't take long before the excitement came to the United States, and that's when I discovered that this kind of experience isn't just fun. It's *sexy.* I'm not just talking about the sort of under-the-table flirting you can really get away with only in a blackout. (At least,

I'm pretty sure I got away with it. But what if the waiters had night-vision goggles? Oh, now I'm embarrassed.) No, I'm talking about the astonishing sensuality of the whole thing. This seduction will arouse more than your sweetie's taste buds.

Tell her not to worry about Saturday night. You're going to prepare a treat for her and take care of *everything.* Ah, those are magic words to a woman. She'll be thrilled to hear them and, more important, she'll be thinking about you all week long. Sometime before the weekend, send her an e-mail: *Dinner on Saturday at 7. Dress code: panties and the biggest, most comfortable T-shirt you own.*

Wow. Her sense of anticipation is off the scale.

Are you a really good cook? Then go for it. Make a masterpiece. But for everyone else, I recommend buying dinner from a great restaurant and taking it home. Avoid spaghetti or anything with sloppy sauces. Steak is fine, but it had better be butter-soft. When picking your menu, try to imagine what it would be like to eat some of it with your fingers. I found a perfect solution at my favorite Greek restaurant: tender baked Athenian chicken that simply falls off the bone, pita bread that gets torn into pieces and dipped in hummus or tangy *tzatziki* sauce, small chunks of feta cheese, finger-sized rolls of grape leaves.

Bring it all home and keep it hidden from your girl as you split it all up onto plates. Turn on

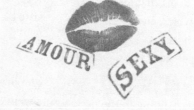
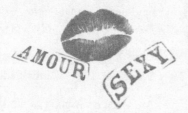
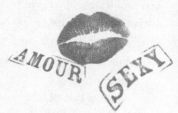

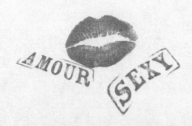

seduction no. 45

Twenty-Two-Point-Five

GREAT BRITAIN

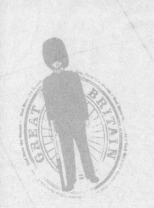

FOR *his* EYES ONLY

$

want to spend some *real* money, go online and be amazed at the range of high-end leather-and-steel gear crafted for serious bondage. Wow. I recommend ribbons because you can get them at any fabric store, cut to different lengths, and they're pretty and festive. Put one on the door and then tie another to the reading lamp on your sweetie's side of the bed. Don't explain. Just let her wonder.

Start your Friday evening with drinks, fun, and romance. When you move to the bedroom and get her undressed, grab your ribbons and give her a wicked grin. Explain your plan for the night. You are going to play with her, and she is going to be unable to resist. Have her lie on her back. Lift her left leg in the air. Ask her for her left hand. Tie her wrist to her ankle with a ribbon. Not tight. You don't want to scare her or cut off her circulation. Now tie her right wrist to her right ankle. *Nice.* She's got her legs in the air, knees slightly bent. It's really quite a comfortable position. And it leaves her bottom completely exposed.

Slide her to the edge of the bed. Ooh! Now there's a surprising thrill for her. Moving her body like that is a show of control. *"What a pretty present, all tied with bows. . . ."* Kneel on the floor before her and begin to work on her with your tongue. Don't hesitate to get physical; grab her calves, open her thighs, press your weight into her. After several minutes, turn her onto her side, facing away from you. Her fantasy of submission is heightened when she can't see your face. Bring out your secret weapon—a vibrator and a bottle of personal lubricant. Cover her whole backside in slippery lube and drive her crazy with the vibe. Let your fingers roam all over her bare behind while you use the toy to draw slow circles around her clit. If she comes, ease up for a few minutes, then begin again. Teach her about the magic of multiple orgasms. Finally, pull her to her knees, butt high, facedown. She'll be glowing with arousal. She may be exhausted, in the best possible way. If you have done your job well, her head will be lost in a land of erotic make-believe, and her vulva will be swollen and wet. That's your cue to make yourself hard and slip yourself into her for a fantasy ride of your own.

Has it been twenty-two and a half minutes yet? Then you're not done.

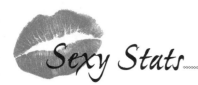

Sexy Stats

- According to *Men's Health*, 89 percent of women who have never had kinky sex think it could improve their sex lives. 93 percent of women who tried kinky sex say it did.

- 43 percent of sexually active adults in the UK own a vibrator.

- British television runs advertisements for "relationship aids," including one that featured a man proposing to a woman with a vibrating "engagement ring."

- In the British Isles, 36 percent of people use ties, rope, or other "riggings" when they sail the sexy seas.

No. 45 TWENTY-TWO-POINT-FIVE

INGREDIENTS
two 24-inch lengths of wide satin ribbon
(or, if you prefer, scarves, soft nylon rope, panty hose, Velcro restraints)
several sticky notes

"There's a good reason why English men are the most sexually satisfied in our survey. They know how to use their mouths. British men aren't afraid to ask for what they want in bed."　　—Men's Health

In the course of doing my research for this book, I came across an astonishing number: *twenty-two-point-five.* That's 22.5 minutes, the longest average amount of time spent on foreplay among all the nations according to *Men's Health* magazine, and that hot global record belongs to . . .

The British. Now, I know what you're thinking: *Is that all? I go* way *longer than that!* Except that, um, you don't. You think you do, but scientists have been watching and timing you.

My own reaction was the *British*? Really? They seem so reserved in the movies. But it turns out that our cousins across the pond are fiends in the sack. On average, they not only spend more time doing the deed, they are also more willing to experiment with it. For one thing, they dress up for it. Just look at those incredible British fetish-wear catalogs. They are also quite comfortable talking about it. And here's another fun surprise. The English lead the world in both vibrator ownership and light bondage. (I'm booking London for my next vacation.)

I didn't know what to make of this next statistic, though. In the United States, it's the woman who is more likely to tie up her man. In England, the lads are most likely to tie the knot. Why is that, do you suppose? I haven't found anyone who can answer that question for me, but I have a guess. I think it might be that English girls, already more open and experienced about sex than most, have discovered the true secret behind bondage: *The one with the restraints is having the most fun.*

Sure, you can get your kicks by being in control. But when you can't move and can't resist, all you really *can* do is focus on sensation. Plus, you're not expected to do any work. With a trustworthy partner, you can sit back (or lie back, or throw your head back while you're tied spread-eagle to the bedposts) and enjoy the ride.

Anticipation makes any act of seduction more fun, so start teasing your sweetie early in the week. Leave a note attached to her steering wheel. It doesn't have to be fancy; a yellow sticky note will do. *Looking forward to a weekend with you*, it says. Sweet, no? Leave another love note on the shower door: *Been thinking about you all week. Love you.* Send her an e-mail with a more direct invitation: *Would love some quiet time with you. How about we shut off the phone and stay in Friday night?* As Friday grows closer, tease her sense of curiosity. Tie a red satin ribbon to the knob of your bedroom door.

It doesn't *have* to be a ribbon. There are so many wonderful things you can use to restrain a lover, and you are free to pick whatever you want, so long as it is soft and flexible and long enough. Scarves are perfect, if a little predictable. The Brits popularized plastic bondage tape, which is very much like the cling wrap you have in your kitchen drawer but in pretty colors. If you want to spend some money, you can find Velcro-backed straps in every adult boutique, and if you

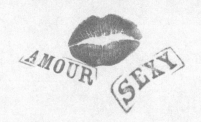
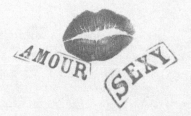

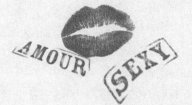
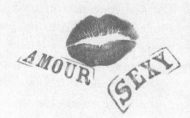
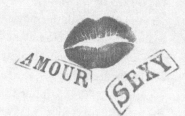
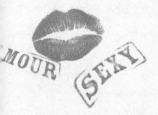

seduction no. 46

Private Screening

ITALY

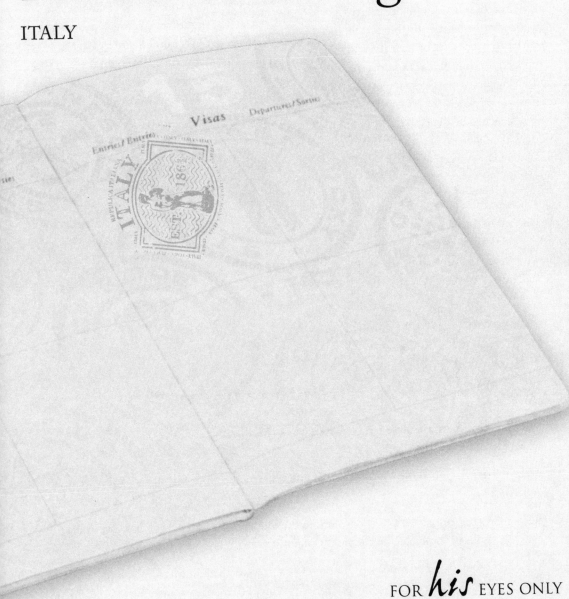

FOR *his* EYES ONLY

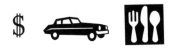

player or a laptop with a couple of movies ready. A blanket and cushions. It's adorable.

Once upon a time, America had something like those Italian love parks, places where couples could have fun and romance without much hassle, and with a bathroom nearby—all that, plus the benefit of a feature film, too. Generations of young lovers first started unzipping by the light of the big screen. A whole lot of couples spent their date nights dry-humping in Technicolor at the drive-in. There aren't many places like that anymore, but you've created one especially for your girl tonight, and she'll be touched by the effort. Ask her to help you tuck the pillowcases over the side windows for a little extra privacy, and then have her snuggle up with you for the show.

Your modern theater has one big advantage over the old ones: *a pause button*. Because there will certainly come a time when the action on the screen is overshadowed by the action in the audience. It starts with a kiss. Then your hands start to slide down her arms, and over her breasts. That moment when your fingers first slip past the buttons of her blouse is always such a turn-on. Go slow at first. Give her time to enjoy the old memories of her early bump-and-grind sessions. Make her feel like a teenager again. Retrace all the steps in her sexual development. When you finally convince her to touch you, down there—and to let you touch her—when you finally get her jeans off and legs apart, calves wrapped around your thighs, right there in the cramped quarters of your car, well, that's just *dirty*. Which is how you know you're doing it right.

Just don't let your Dad catch you. You will be *so* grounded.

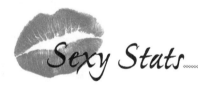

Sexy Stats

- The first drive-in movie played in New Jersey in 1933. It was called *Wife Beware*. Beware of what? The stick shift?

- *Molto romantico*: Italian men ask if they can kiss you, whether your first date or your twentieth anniversary.

- Risky behaviors cause a rush of endorphins in the brain, which may explain why sex in the backseat thrills us so much. The possibility of getting caught is a huge turn-on.

- The quintessential *Italian stallion*—Giacomo Casanova—actually wasn't so much to look at, yet women fell at his feet. Why? He put it best, saying, "To make a woman feel special, do something special." Yep. What *he* said.

- Dry humping isn't just for horny teenagers. Rubbing up against your partner while clothed creates friction, making you both wildly turned on. Your brains will associate it with the frustrated make-out sessions of your youth.

INGREDIENTS

1 car
1 portable DVD player or laptop
2 drinks and snacks

1 blindfold (bandanna or scarf)
2 movies
2 pillowcases

I USED TO *LOVE* MAKING OUT IN A CAR. SOME of my hottest memories involve automobiles, and boys, and more sweat than a young lady is supposed to have. Part of what makes car sex so awesome, of course, is the sheer difficulty of having it. One of the great lessons of love is that passion is always enhanced by obstacles.

And a car has *plenty* of those. (Once I actually got stuck under the steering wheel!) That's why I was so tickled by Europe's latest innovation in automotive arousal. Italians can now get their groove on in "love parks"—parking lots created specifically for couples who want to steam up the windows. In return for your hourly rental fee, you get a little privacy, with walls or screens between parking spaces, and a little security. But this business isn't built on nostalgia. It's based on necessity. A lot of Italians do it in their cars because the alternative is to do it at home. With *madre e padre* in the next room. *Mamma mia!*

And that's the flip side of those famously close Italian families. A surprisingly high percentage of young Italian men live at home into their thirties, and if they want to go lock lips with their *ragazzaes*, well, their only choices are front seat or backseat. This is not so much a handicap as it is a training ground. If you can get a woman aroused in a car—if you can get her *off* while her clothes are still *on*—then you are a very skilled lover, indeed. These *uomini italiani* aren't just coasting on the legend of Casanova, you know;

they have earned their reputations as hot lovers. And they have the automobile to thank for it.

This week, you're going to re-create a *molto sexy* car fantasy, with an old-fashioned American twist. As always, start by tweaking your sweetie's sense of curiosity. Send her an e-mail: *Special date on Saturday night! I'll take care of everything. Casual dress. You bring two pillowcases.*

Pillowcases? Okay, you got her attention with that one. She'll spend the whole week smiling and wondering what you're up to. (And telling her girlfriends about it. They will be envious, of course.) When Saturday rolls around, tell her to take the pillowcases and get into the car. (Bonus option for big spenders: rent a car! Ooh, make it an *Italian* car. So sexy.) Go for a drive—anywhere will do—and after ten minutes or so, pull over and ask her to open the glove box. There's a scarf inside. And in order to prepare for your big surprise, she has to use it to cover her eyes. Once she's blindfolded, give her a kiss and then start driving to your destination. Which might be a special romantic spot, a lover's lane . . . or your very own driveway.

Keep talking to her while you get your accessories out of the trunk and set up inside the car. When you're ready, tell her to take off the blindfold and have a look. She'll be amazed at what you've done. Right there, in the backseat, you've created the twenty-first-century version of a *drive-in theater*. Sodas and snacks. A DVD

seduction no. 47

Meet Me in Paradise

HAWAII

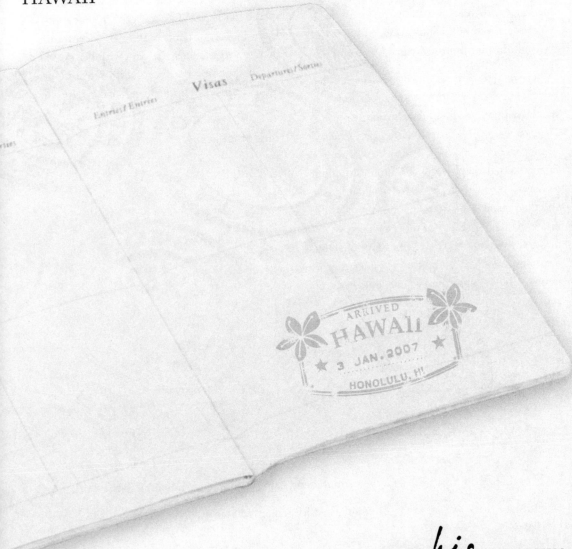

FOR *his* EYES ONLY

to her buttock and down again. Repeat on her other leg.

When you've finished the backs of her legs, help her flip over (she'll be *flippin'* slippery!) and work from her neck to her legs, slowly and gently massaging anything that isn't covered by her bathing suit. *Super slo-mo* is the name of the game. You need only about fifteen minutes, but you can never have too much. It should feel like you're moving at a snail's pace. Focus on her needs. Be mindful and caring, and that will transmit through your massage.

When you get to the fronts of her legs, let your fingers linger on her inner thighs. Let your hands "happen" to slip under the elastic once ("*Excuse me, miss!*"), twice ("*I apologize, it won't happen again!*"), and on the third pass, turn your fingers so that they graze her mound, stopping to hover over her hole, just barely touching her, and then resume the massage on her leg. You'll know when she's ready for more by the little noises she makes and the way her hips push up into your fingers. Watch for tents under your sarong, *keiki*, because the two coconuts between your legs are about to get a serious milking.

Bend down and whisper, *"Let's continue this in your cabana."* Help her to stand and lead her inside, bringing the CD player with you. Help her out of her suit and lower her to the bed. Let your sarong drop while you make out with your girl. Continue where you left off outside, but this time without the pesky suit in your way.

Slowly massage from her inner thighs to her lower lips and circle her clit with your fingers. Spread her legs and kneel between them with the head of your penis waiting at her entrance. Then, when she's begging you with her eyes and mouth, grabbing the sheets and your head, dive into her until you both smell like coconut—like *summer*.

Hang ten, *Kahuna*.

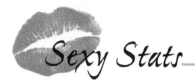 Sexy Stats

- Hawaiian Tropic, with its famous coconut scent, is the #1 brand of suntan oil in the world.
- Outdoor massages are the most popular service requested at upscale hotels on the Hawaiian islands.
- For sex on the beach, doggie style is the most popular (and sand-free) position.
- Studies have linked higher levels of testosterone to men who live in warm climates.

No. 47 MEET ME IN PARADISE

INGREDIENTS
deck chair cushions or an inflatable pool lounge
1 portable CD or MP3 player
1 outdoor spot in the shade

several large towels
1 CD of surf sounds or Hawaiian ballads
coconut-scented suntan oil

In Hawaii the tourism industry is focused on one thing: bringing the visitors as much relaxation as possible, while making them feel like royalty. It's time for the truth now, boys. We ladies like to be catered to. We may not be used to it, but we like it very much.

And I can tell you, the people of Hawaii have the catering bit down to a science. Not only do we get *lei'd* when we arrive at the airport, but at the resort I stayed at, cabana boys were there to bring drinks and food, and to offer massages as I lay on the beach. This seduction practically guarantees that your lady will be swept away by you, her cabana boy. Setting the scene is most of the work, though, and big effort earns big payoffs.

E-mail her a sexy tropical photo. Include a note saying, *Meet me in Paradise, Saturday, 4 P.M.* If you share a computer, download a Hawaiian beach screen saver. She's going to smile all week wondering what you've got planned.

She's not allowed to watch while you prepare a spot outdoors (your backyard or patio is great) for her Hawaiian getaway. Set up the cushions on the ground and cover with a towel. Place your coconut-scented oil in a spot of sunshine so it's nice and warm for her. Play some nature sounds of the surf, or if you're going for authenticity, traditional Hawaiian ballads. I'm talking Keali 'i Reichel's CD, *Kamahiwa*. Trust me on this.

Now, get your music or surf sounds going, provide a cool drink (a piña colada or a mai tai would be good; don't forget the little umbrella!), and wrap something comfortable like a towel (or a sarong, if you're channeling David Beckham—hot!) around your waist. Then tell your lady that her massage will take place outdoors and to please change into her bathing suit.

Meet her outside, with her drink in your hand, and let her take in the sight and sound of your little oasis. Seeing you in your sarong, ready to attend to her, with the sounds of the islands softly playing will make her smile and say, *"Awww!"* Kiss her and say, *"Welcome to Hawaii, miss. Would you lie facedown, please?"* For the next fifteen minutes, do not speak.

Kneel at her head, spread some oil on your palms, and glide your hands down the center of her back and up the sides. Use enough pressure not to tickle but not enough to cause pain; this is a seduction, after all! Breathe slowly, which will signal to her that she should relax and breathe deeply.

She'll inhale the scent of coconut, imagining your Hawaiian vacation together, as your hands stroke her back, shoulders, and neck smoothly and slowly. Move to her side and spread more oil on her legs in an upward direction. Let your fingers travel underneath the elastic of her bikini bottom a couple times before sliding it over to expose her cheek. Continue from her thigh up

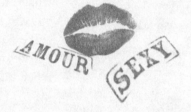

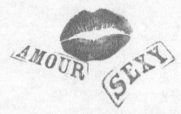

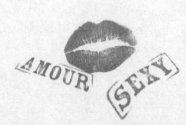

seduction no. **48**

Hot Step

ARGENTINA

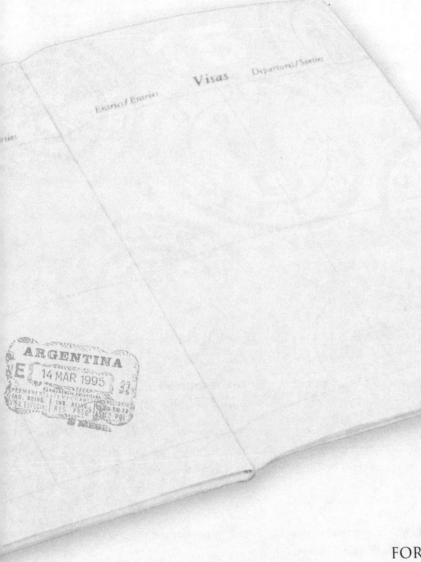

FOR *his* EYES ONLY

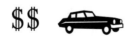

this dance? Keep the dance theme going over the next couple of days, taking her in your arms at random times and twirling her around the house. Finally, ask her out for a date—and tell her to wear her dancing shoes.

She will be *thrilled*. And she'll be tickled when you pull up in front of a dance studio. That first session will probably be slightly less elegant than Brad and Angelina, but you'll score a lot of points with her just for trying and end up with lots to laugh about in bed. Stick with it, though, and the real nature of the tango will start to show through. You see, it's the man who does the driving on this dance. With nothing but your right hand, a little confidence, and those basic eight steps, you control everything she does. You dominate. You look totally cool while you're doing it.

Even better, you make *her* look good and feel sexy. And that's a skill that always pays off, whether you're dancing vertically . . . or not.

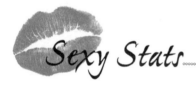

Sexy Stats

- The tango originated in bordellos. Sort of a test drive, I guess. The 1890s version of the lap dance.

- Women can't help being attracted to a man who knows how to shake his hips. Science has measured the increase in sex chemicals in the brains of women watching guys on the dance floor.

- Visit Argentina today and you'll hear and see everything tango permeating Buenos Aires. Walk down any street in the city and you can sample tango art and history. There is a twenty-four-hour tango TV channel, tango dancers on the streets, two tango clubs per block, curios and postcards, and even an altar to Carlos Gardel, a prominent originator and singer of Argentine tango.

- Latin dances like the Tango Merengue, and *Paso Doble* are consistently the most popular dances at studios across the country with men and women.

- Argentine tango is improvisational and unpredictable, similar to a puzzle that gets put together differently each time. There are no real "steps" in Argentine tango, but a walk forward, back, and sideways. The man leads with his mind and body, and the woman follows with hers.

No. 48 HOT STEP

INGREDIENTS
1 movie with a tango
1 or more tango lessons
2 polished shoes

SEAN CONNERY DID IT. SO DID ARNOLD Schwarzenegger and Robert Duvall and Brad Pitt. Richard Gere did it so well he was asked to come back and do it again.

Al Pacino? He's so cool he did it *blind*. Hoo-ah!

They all danced the tango in movies.

And they were *awesome*. Powerful, sexual, and totally masculine. They made a hundred million women go all tingly in the pudenda. That's because the tango is, at its heart, a seduction. That's not a metaphor. The tango is not a *stylized* seduction, or a *ritualized representation* of a seduction. It's the real thing: man, woman, hooking up on a dance floor.

I'm not talking about the competition version of the tango. That's just for show. I loved watching *Dancing With the Stars*, but what you're seeing there is ballroom tango, about as real as reality TV. The genuine article is, um, dirtier. It's loaded with passion. It's about getting so close to your partner that you can feel her heartbeat. It's an embrace so sensual that she wraps her arms *and a leg* around you. The tango is *sex standing up*, eight hot steps at a time. (And often with strangers!)

You'll find *milongueros*—skilled, devoted tango dancers—gathering weekly in major cities all over the world. And the ones who get really serious, more than half a million every year, eventually make their way to Buenos Aires, the mecca of tango. You could spend your entire vacation, or your entire life, pursuing passion on the dance floors of Argentina. Lots of people do. So consider yourself warned about this week's seduction: *Your first hit could get you hooked*.

Well, maybe not your *very* first hit. In fact, the first time you step on the floor with an instructor, you are probably going to feel clumsy. Those eight basic steps—backward, to the side, a few forward, to the side again—have to be memorized. But here's why it's worth it: *Your woman wants you to take control of her*. Not all the time; of course not. But for a few minutes, or a few hours, every woman wants to indulge in the fantasy of being pursued and captured. The tango is a romance novel come to life, where the headstrong heroine finally meets a man worthy of her submission. Catch her on the dance floor, and she will be yours in the bedroom.

It would be fun to start your seduction with a movie, just to get your baby in the mood. You can't go wrong with Pacino's classic *Scent of a Woman*, but for a bit more action—tango with guns and knives!—check out Brad and Angelina in *Mr. & Mrs. Smith*. Richard Gere's *Shall We Dance* is pure chick flick, but if you don't mind subtitles, the original Japanese version is better. And I have to recommend a personal favorite, a sweet, funny Aussie film from the nineties called *Strictly Ballroom*.

Rent one and watch it with your sweetie. The next day, send her a text message: *May I have*

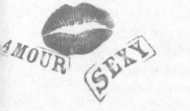

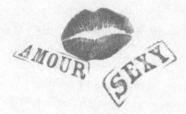
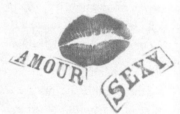

seduction no. 49

Always Look Back

BRAZIL

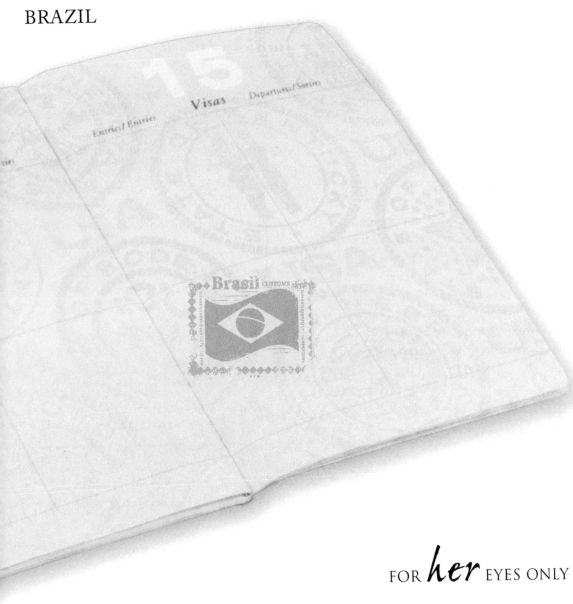

FOR *her* EYES ONLY

Most important, start drawing attention to your bottom in positive ways. Don't ever say, "Honey, do these pants make my ass look fat?" (Very old punch line: *"No, of course not. It's those double cheeseburgers that make your ass look fat!"* Heh.) Try this instead: *"Hey, these new pants make my ass look pretty great, don't they?"* Walk across the room in front of him, smack your bottom, and proudly proclaim, *"I know you like that!"* Give him a wink and a wiggle as you walk away. Do something like that every single day. This isn't just look-on-the-bright-side wishful thinking. This is *advertising*. Spend a week telling him how good you feel about your backside, and he will start to notice it, too. He'll start to believe it. He'll start to look forward to its every appearance.

Oh, and what an appearance it's going to make. Saturday night, set your honey up in a comfortable chair and tell him to get ready for a show. Hit the music. Dash into the next room and whip off the skirt you had over your costume. Now enter the room, back end first. Put your cheeks through the door and shimmy. Dance closer to him, bottom first, and let him admire your cheeks, hanging out of your snug boy shorts. Encourage audience participation;

have him tug the shorts off to reveal your new pretty panties. And after a while, let him see the layer hiding under that. It is *awesome*. You are wearing a thong, the kind with a beautiful decoration where the straps all come together in back, right above your butt crack. A feather? A jewel? A metal clasp? Oh, there are hundreds of crazy-sexy styles to choose from, and it almost doesn't matter which one you pick, because they all have the power to hypnotize a man. Snuggle into his lap; use the might of your magnificent cheeks to get him aroused.

Finally, lead him to the bedroom for the final act of your show. He gets to lie on the bed while you kneel next to him. Your attention, and your mouth, are focused on his penis. But *his* attention will be drawn elsewhere. That's because you have arranged things so that a mirror is in precisely the right position to give him the view he craves. His eyes will be glued to your rear. You might still imagine you have a butt-full of flaws.

But your guy is a Brazilian now. And all he sees is *perfeição*—sheer, flawless perfection.

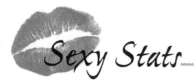

Sexy Stats

- The butt culture of Brazil exploded in the 1970s with the string bikini. The latest trend in bottom baring? Stick-on pubikinis and bikinis with strings so thin they're called *fio dental*. Yep, dental floss.

- In 1993, Sir Mix-a-Lot won a Grammy for his song "Baby Got Back," now an anthem for connoisseurs of the derriere: *Don't want none unless you got buns, hun!*

- G-strings have been used by exotic dancers and burlesque performers since the 1920s. Burlesque legend Gypsy Rose Lee even wrote a novel called *The G-String Murders*.

- Samba dancers at Carnavale wear outrageously high heels, which accentuate their already voluptuous behinds.

No. 49 ALWAYS LOOK BACK

INGREDIENTS
1 fancy thong
1 pair of pretty panties
1 pair of sexy boy shorts
1 bedroom mirror
hot music

WANT TO FEEL BETTER ABOUT YOUR BOTTOM? Go to Brazil.

"Whoa, hold on, Corn," I hear you say. "Isn't Brazil the world capital of magnificent asses? Isn't Carnavale where all the great tushes come from? Are you suggesting that I might feel better about my own jiggly butt by going to the homeland of *Gisele Bündchen?*"

Yes, I am. And here's why. Park yourself on a Brazilian beach and watch the girls walk by. Do they all have perfect butts? No. In fact, you're going to see big butts and tiny butts, skinny butts and sagging butts. Some are way past their prime, and some look like two bags of packing peanuts. And sure, some look like Gisele. But what these women have in common is that *they all clearly love their butts*! They stroll around in short dresses, tiny shorts, and bikinis so small that they had to invent the Brazilian wax job. (Speaking of which, I'll bet you didn't even know you had hair way back there. Well, you do, and if you're going to wear a Brazilian thong, you should really do something about that. It doesn't hurt, not *at all*.)

The buttastic confidence of Brazilian women rubbed off on me as I was researching this book. I began to look at my own bumbum in a new light. Instead of being mildly embarrassed by it, I made myself speak highly of it, at least around the house. Instead of dressing to hide it, I found ways to show it off. (Thank you, Frankie B!) And suddenly, I noticed that Jeff was admiring

it much more. He complimented my butt and grabbed it. I caught other men staring at it. It was the same ass I always had except, sadly, getting dramatically older every year, but it seemed to be drawing more love and affection than ever.

I talked with my girlfriends about it and discovered that one of my dearest companions has a whole heinie thing going on with her husband that can be summarized thusly: *He adores her butt.* Worships it. I've never seen her bottom, so all I can say is that it, um, seems nice, but she apparently parades it around the house like a Nascar trophy because it makes him wild.

That's when it hit me. *We can all be Brazilians.* It doesn't take a perfect rear. It just takes confidence. Plus a close shave. And some tiny, tiny underwear.

While shopping for your *new* underwear, use some of your old stuff for bait. That is, leave some of your panties in surprising places for your guy to find. Hang your undies from his rearview (get it?) mirror. Stuff a pair into his laptop bag. Put some in his underwear drawer. Hide a pair in his pocket for a workplace surprise. In the meantime, begin showing a little more rear cleavage around the house. Wear your low-rise jeans and bend over right in front of him. Prance around in panties. Put on your shortest skirt and let him catch several glimpses of that magic line where your cheeks meet your thighs.

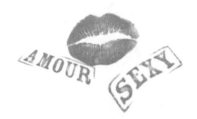

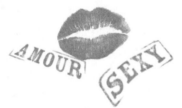
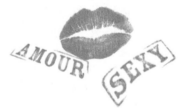
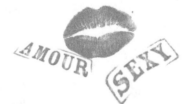
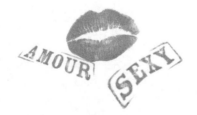
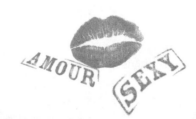

seduction no. **50**

The Kitty Triangle

CULTURAL COCKTAIL: INDIA, CHINA

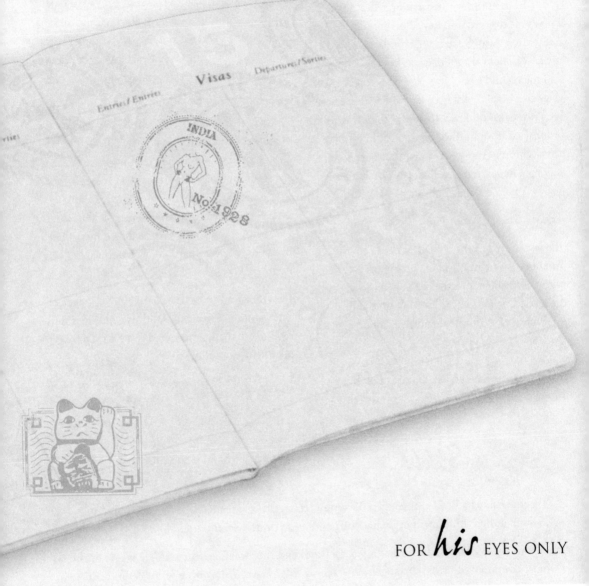

FOR *his* EYES ONLY

from the goddess Shakti herself. *Take your time.* Visit each tip of the triangle with your lips and fingertips, slowly getting more aggressive as you feel her body warm beneath you.

The next triangle is formed by her clitoris and her feet.

Ahh, the feet—so sadly neglected by most men and so in need of loving attention. Rub them. Press your thumbs into her soles and massage her tension away. Squeeze her ankles and the muscles in her calves. Focus on her toes, tugging and rolling and stretching each one. A foot rub is an awesome experience, and here's why: Those long nerves take a little detour on their way to the brain, passing right through the neighborhood of the clitoris. And when those foot nerves start singing a happy song, well, the clit hears them and just can't help but join right in.

And it's time for you to join the fun.

The last triangle is the one that connects the other two, the Kitty Triangle, from breasts to vagina, from nips to lips, and you get to visit all the angles over and over, turning up the heat every time you complete another circuit.

By now you've put the better part of an hour into playing with your mate. And she's felt your love and attention, literally from head to toe. True Tantricas would try to stay right there for the rest of the night, balanced on that incredible buzz right before climax. But that's a lesson for another day. Right now, it's your job to bring her over the top, focusing all your attention on her clit, spinning slow circles around it with your tongue, warming it with your breath, trapping it with your lips. Go faster. Get stronger. Pin her to the bed; let her feel your Shiva strength while you pour your energy into her pleasure. Bring her to ecstasy and, like the young Tantra students of four thousand years ago, get ready to drink the nectar of your goddess.

Massaging your feet benefits your overall health. A form of reflexology, foot massage is based on the idea that your whole body is reflected in your foot. Experts claim this type of massage reduces stress and induces relaxation. And it feels *so* good. The *Kama Sutra* contains great advice about giving oral sex to your sweetie. The celebrated love text advises you to "pinch the arched lips of her house of love very, very slowly together, and kiss them as though you kissed her lower lip."

Don't forget her hands. Along with the feet, they contain seven thousand two hundred nerve endings that are considered to be a road map to her entire body.

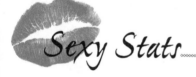

- Tibetan scholars have a timeless philosophy: The triad of a sexual relationship is based on looking at her, thinking about what you're going to do to her, and then doing it.

- **tri • an • gle** Along with the landing strip (line) and the Brazilian, the triangle is one of three most common pubic hair arrangements a female can have. *The triangle points downward toward the clit. (Urban Dictionary)*

- Proving once and for all that the carpet doesn't necessarily need to match the drapes, the Betty Beauty company manufactures hair dye for the hair *down there.* In 2007 the company sold 75,000 boxes of its most popular product: a hot pink dye called Fun Betty.

No. 50 THE KITTY TRIANGLE

INGREDIENTS
sticky notes
your girl
patience and dedication

EASTERN PHILOSOPHY AND RELIGIONS HAVE a following here in the West, but their growth has been hampered by the fact that they can be hard to explain. Tantra, for example, has a history that goes back more than 4,000 years, and these days it's splintered into lots of different styles and interpretations. But I think a whole lot more Americans would dive into tantra if they understood this one core principle:

The girl's gotta come!

Okay, I might be oversimplifying. But tantric sex is almost the *opposite* of religions that say sex is not for pleasure. Done right (with techniques that can make it last for hours), Tantric sex is considered a doorway to the divine. Think of that the next time you get down on your knees.

But here's the part that really made me smile. In Tantra's earliest forms, the sharing of body fluids was a sacrament. A young initiate was expected to partake of the juice of an aroused woman. Scholars might hem and haw when describing that in their textbooks, but dude, that is *oral sex* they're talking about! In the old days, when you joined the club, you had to go down on the Woman in Charge. (Can I get an *amen*!) There's more to it, of course, but couples that practice Tantra today spend a *lot* of time tapping in to their sexual energy.

This week you're going to crank up your mate's sexual energy with a recipe that's part Tantra and part *Kama Sutra*, with a dash of reflexology and a light, sweet coating of Corn. Sex is always more fun when you give your mate some time to think about it in advance, so tease her early in the week with a handful of Post-it notes. Put one on her steering wheel and one on her bathroom mirror. Put one on the fridge and one on her purse. Everywhere she goes this week, she should find cute little notes that have one of the following things on them:

three triangles, like this:
a heart ❤
the words *Bedroom. Saturday. 7 P.M. Love you!*

Triangles? Yes, that's right. They add to the anticipation, because she'll be wondering all week long about your upcoming surprise. These three triangles, form a diagram of the most sensitive parts of her body, like a map of her erogenous zones. A map you get to follow Saturday night.

Tantric sex isn't slow so much as it is *long,* to give you both time to enjoy each delicious step on the path to orgasm.

The first triangle for you to focus on is the one formed by her mouth and her nipples.

MOUTH

NIPPLES

Less enlightened men might just twirl her nipples like radio dials while tongue wrestling her tonsils, but with your raised tantric consciousness, you know how to tease her with gentle kisses and soft caresses. You know how to play with her breasts before they are bare and how to undress them as if they were a gift

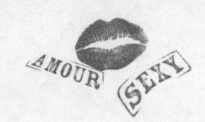

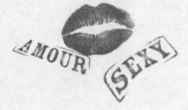

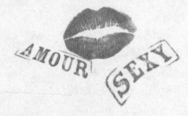
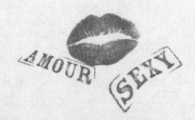

seduction no. 51

Let The Games Begin

GREECE

FOR *his* EYES ONLY

$

you're going to do. *You're going to challenge her.* Make it a game, a competition between the two of you.

Send her an e-mail with the rules of the game: *Put on four pieces of clothing tonight. No more. Before the night is over, you'll be naked. Why? Because we're going to play a game. A competition. What is it? I can't tell! But you're going to love it. Guaranteed. All you need to know is this: Something is going to happen that will make you so hot you'll want to take off your clothes. But it's up to you. You'll be in charge. P.S. I'll be wearing four pieces of clothing, too.*

She'll be so curious she'll shoot you back an e-mail, *begging* to know what you have planned. Tease her a little more with a second e-mail: *Okay, honey, here's the deal for tonight: Every fifteen minutes, I'm going to surprise you. BUT to get your surprise, you have to remove a piece of clothing. I'll take off a piece of clothing, too . . . if you accept all my challenges, you guessed it. At the end of an hour, we'll both be nude!*

Cool, huh? But what are you going to surprise her with? How about gifts? *What can you give her to make her take off her clothes?*—you ask. Remember the Greeks and the Trojan horse? It was a gift from the Greeks to the Trojans, but with a big surprise inside: soldiers. You're going to give her gifts with a big surprise at the end: *you!*

You can charm your gal if your gift-giving approach is more sentimental than materialistic. Ever try to read a woman's body lingo when she gets a gift? Something that tugs at her heart strings works every time: A fresh flower picked from the garden, a smooth rock with *I love you* painted on it, her favorite magazine, massage oil, or decadent chocolate will melt her clothes off her faster than you can say, "Twist 'n' shout." And that's the last gift: a Twister game—your own personal nude Olympics.

Don't forget: Keep the gifts a secret. This is important because the *last* gift is behind closed doors. Challenge her to take off her last piece of clothing by telling her *where* the gift is (make sure the room or space is large enough for the mat). Her imagination will run wild. She'll be *dying* to know what it is and will do *anything* to find out, but keep her in suspense. Make her *squirm* before you open the door.

When she rushes through the door with you right behind her, make sure the game is set up, iced drinks ready, and fun music playing. Then challenge her to a game of Naked Twister. You'll be amazed how quickly she'll lose herself in the game.

This is one game where you'll *both* score the winning point!

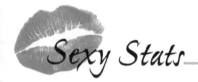

Sexy Stats

- Women who engage regularly in physical exercise (Naked Twister, anyone?) reach a state of arousal more quickly, enjoy the benefits of a stronger libido, *and* are so in touch with their bodies they can climax in a shorter time.

- The Twister game was patented in 1966 and became controversial when competitors deemed it "sex in a box" because the game required players to use their bodies as game pieces.

$\mathcal{N}o.$ *51* LET THE GAMES BEGIN

INGREDIENTS
stopwatch
game of Twister
4 small gifts (flowers, costume jewelry, chocolate, massage oil, erotic novel, vibrator or dildo)

THERE'S NOTHING THAT TURNS ME ON MORE than a hunky, muscular guy ripping off his shirt during a neighborhood football game, his bare chest glistening with sweat and making this sun goddess ache with desire. "*Too bad men don't play sports in the nude,*" I said to a friend of mine as we walked along the beach on a hot, humid day and a guy jogged by, his cute butt working it, the muscles on his bare chest pumping and grinding. She whispered to me that in ancient Greece athletes competed nude in the Olympic Games.

No loincloth? A mischievous grin lit up my face as I imagined the jogging stud sans shorts.

She shook her head and smiled. Zilch, zero, nada.

I couldn't wait to jump on the Internet and check this out. Here's the deal: Not only did men perform all sports activities in the nude in ancient Greece, but women removed their clothes whenever the whim pleased them. Of course, it was hard to be shy in a society where the naked human form was on public display everywhere in the form of statues and phallic symbols, and masturbation was considered a gift of the gods.

Who knew ancient Greece was one big happy nudist camp?

It didn't take me long to whip this seduction into shape. All I could think about were nude bodies, ancient dildos, and men and women hungering

for each other. But it's going to take some doing on *your* part to make your girl comfortable in the buff, which means you'll have to also shed *your* duds when she does.

Are you up to the challenge?

I've no doubt your male machinery will be up to just about *anything* when her first piece of clothing comes off. But we've got to make *her* comfortable with the seduction, so you're going to take it nice and easy and show her how much fun it is to be nude. It worked for the Greeks and it can work for you.

This is your chance to be a Greek God and free yourself from the rigors of clothing as the ancient Greeks did for an evening with the love of your life. Flirt, play, tease each other, but the goal is for both of you to strip down to nothing while you go about your business within the privacy of your home. Read the newspaper, go on the Internet, talk on your cell phone, prepare a meal, or play an indoor sport. All in the nude. But just like the Olympics, there are rules: You can't touch her and she can't touch you until the time you set beforehand.

So how are you going to get her to take off her clothes? When you ask a woman what she likes about herself, she'll answer her eyes, her smile, her long hair, but women rarely mention a body part. They never think their bodies are perfect enough, but you love her just the way she is. You've got to convince *her* of that. So here's what

seduction no. 52

The Laura Corn
Challenge

UNITED STATES

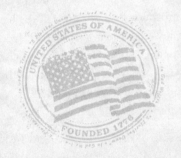

FOR *his* EYES ONLY

$$$

Velcro cuff—*ziiiip*—and fasten it gently around her wrist. She *definitely* wasn't expecting this. Kiss her again.

Move to the other side and whisper in her other ear, *"I'm going to take good care of you. I love you so much."* On goes the second wrist strap.

Position the straps slowly; there's nothing like a long pause followed by the sound of Velcro pulling apart to heighten the anticipation. She's going to be putty in your firm but gentle hands.

Secure her legs in the ankle restraints, with enough slack for her to bend her knees. Once she's all ready, give her a few moments to pull on the straps. She's thinking—desperately curious—wondering what could possibly happen next.

Begin by exploring her uncharted erogenous zones. Kiss her gently on her neck, just under her jaw. Build up to a lick, and then a suck . . . not enough to leave a mark, but she doesn't know that. Move to another spot, but keep coming back again until she's gasping with pleasure.

Trace her collarbone and down the side of her breast to the ribs—just under her arm—another neglected erogenous zone. Soft kisses and touches there will send shivers through her entire body, and you know where they lead. Your baby's clitoris is just a few inches away, but you're not going there yet.

Stop on your way to her honey pot, at the soft place between hip bone and mound—and here you're *going* to leave a mark. Kiss that spot, suck the flesh into your mouth and hold it there. Leave a red mark, one that will last for days and send her mind flashing back to this moment every time she sees it. *Now* you're ready to give her what she craves: a release of the tension that's been building inside her since she read your note in the bath.

Hover your lips over her clit, barely touching it. Tease it with your tongue while you finger her kitty, inserting two fingers and massaging her G-Spot. Her entire body is on fire, and you know exactly what she needs.

Bring her to orgasm with your mouth and fingers. Kiss her and whisper, *"I need to be inside you."* Leave the restraints and blindfold on. Watch her face and body while you make love, and just before you come, uncover her eyes.

It takes a true adventurer to step outside the safety of what he knows, to accept the Challenge and discover what lies just beyond his everyday boundaries. Your lover will look at you differently, with fresh eyes, as she realizes what's just happened: You've done something unpredictable—taken a *risk*—and to a woman, that is *so* hot.

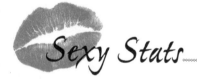

Sexy Stats

- The lips have the highest concentration of nerve endings per centimeter than any other place on the body.

- Women have lots of sexual fantasies, the most popular by far is for a man to take control in the bedroom, adding a few unexpected kinky touches.

- Ladies who enjoy being bound say that it's the feeling of security, rather than the loss of control, that turns them on.

- **chal • lenge** a demanding or stimulating situation. (Urban Dictionary)

No. 52 THE LAURA CORN CHALLENGE

INGREDIENTS
blindfold
under-the-bed restraints
a single rose
an adventurous spirit

WHAT DO WOMEN REALLY WANT? ACCORDING to almost every sex survey ever taken, it's more adventurous men.

I'm not talking about hiking the Appalachian Trail or climbing Mt. Everest; we want our men to be more adventurous *sexually*. This week, your challenge is to break out of your comfort zone. Do something neither of you might ever *think* of doing. You will surprise your sweetie with a night she won't forget for a long, long time.

It centers around one item, hidden from her view, and it's going to make her heart jump, her mind race and her body shiver with anticipation. In fact, when the evening is over, you'll be the undisputed champion of sexual adventure. Every adventurer needs good equipment, and your special piece is a set of under-the-bed restraints.

You can find them online for less than the cost of a night out on the town, and trust me: They may be the best investment you'll ever make, since you'll use them for years in dozens of ways, and they never wear out.

On the night of your date, start building your girl's anticipation by drawing a bath and setting her favorite drink on the edge of the tub. Propped against the glass is an envelope with the words *Open Me*. Inside is a blindfold and a card that reads:

Enjoy your relaxing bath and meet me in our bedroom. Bring the blindfold. Don't worry, I'll make the bed later. Love, Bill

You do realize that "Bill" is you, right??

You've just piqued her curiosity, and her mind has started buzzing. While she soaks in the bath and sips her drink she'll be wondering what *you're* doing in the bedroom.

Take everything off the bed except the bottom sheet, and position the restraints under the mattress. Lay the rose in the center of the bed and light a candle on the nightstand.

After her bath, lead her to the bed. She'll see the nearly bare mattress and the rose and her heart will jump.

Drop her towel to the floor and blindfold her. Her pulse will quicken immediately. Take her hand, *"Baby, I love you."* Slide onto the bed together. Let her get used to the blindfold. With her sight gone, her other senses will be heightened, and that's just what you want.

Lie next to her and tell her how beautiful she looks. Kiss and touch her. Then take the rose and brush it across her lips, letting her inhale its scent. Use the petals to lightly trace the curve of her neck, her breasts, hips and belly.

Seduce her with soft kisses as you trace her body with the rose, ending at her clit. The sensation of a dozen rose petals—like little tongues—circling her bud will drive her wild.

Bring one of the wrist restraints up to the mattress and whisper into that ear, *"I love the way you look when I'm touching you."* Separate the

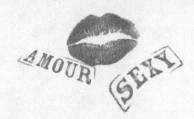

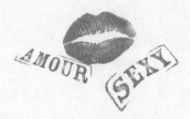
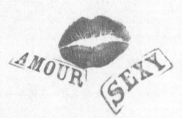
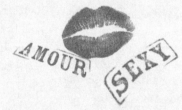
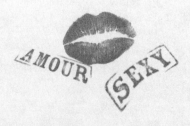

Research Contributors

I want to thank the following people for their valuable help to me in researching this book.

MADELINE GLASS never planned on being a writer of erotica. Her website MadelineintheMirror.com began as a dating-after-divorce journal in 2005 and has been featured on Playboy Radio, Sexoteric.com, and Fleshbot.com. She is a regular contributor to Fleshbot's Sex Blog Roundup and thinks that the Internet can save the world, if you are nice to people. Her sexy writing appears in the anthology *Spanked: Red-Cheeked Erotica* (Cleis Press), and her book of 365 real and deliciously photographed sex positions, *The Daily Kama Sutra*, will be published in 2009. Madeline enjoys coloring outside the lines, eating, and masturbation, usually not all at once.

JINA BACARR loves adventure in exotic locales, which led her to write the RIO award-winning erotic novel, *The Blonde Geisha* (the only erotic novel to win the top spot in Mainstream Fiction), as well as the award-winning nonfiction book, *The Japanese Art of Sex*. She worked as the Japanese consultant on KCBS-TV, MSNBC, TechTV's *Wired for Sex*, Canada's *The Pleasure Zone*, British Sky Broadcasting's *Saucy TV*, La Biennale Arts Festival in Venice, Italy, *Men's Health Guide to the Best Sex in the World* for Rodale Press and *69 Sexy Things 2 Do Before You Die* for Playboy TV. She's the author of Spies, Lies & Naked Thighs and Cleopatra's Perfume.

EDEN BRADLEY writes dark, edgy erotic fiction. Her work has been called "elegant, intelligent and sensual." The author of a number of novels, novellas, and short stories, Eden writes contemporary erotic fiction for Bantam, Berkley, Harlequin Spice Briefs and Phaze Publishing, and her work has appeared in *Cosmopolitan* magazine.

Eden has appeared on Playboy Radio's Night Calls, and conducts workshops on writing sex. When she's not writing, you can find her wandering museums, shopping for shoes and reading everything she can get her hands on. A California native, Eden currently lives in Los Angeles. You can visit her website at www.edenbradley.com.

RACHEL KRAMER BUSSEL (www.rachelkramerbussel.com) is an author, editor, blogger, reading series host, and spanking fan. Her books include *Tasting Him, Tasting Her, Spanked: Red-Cheeked Erotica, Naughty Spanking Stories from A to Z 1* and *2, He's on Top, She's on Top, Caught Looking, Hide and Seek, Dirty Girls,* and the nonfiction anthologies *Best Sex Writing 2008* and *2009.* Her writing has been published in over 100 anthologies, including *Best American Erotica 2004* and *2006, Single State of the Union, Desire: Women Write About Wanting* and *Everything You Know About Sex is Wrong.* She's contributed to *AVN, Bust, Cosmopolitan,* Fresh Yarn, Gothamist, Huffington Post, Mediabistro, *New York Post,* Penthouse, Playgirl, Radar, San Francisco Chronicle, Tango, Thefrisky.com, *Time Out New York,* and other publications. She serves as Senior Editor at *Penthouse Variations,* hosts and curates In The Flesh Erotic Reading Series and wrote the popular Lusty Lady column for *The Village Voice.*

PATRICIA CIHODARU is a thirty-four-year-old Romanian psychologist & psychotherapist, M.D., the chief redactor of a holistic lifestyle magazine named *Body Mind Spirit Magazine,* and collaborator to the Romanian edition of *Men's Health* magazine. She also works in a private clinic in Bucharest as a psychotherapist specializing in cognitive-behavioral therapy; she is coauthor of three books in the psychology field; she translated several personal development books including *Multiorgasmic Couple* by Mantak Chia and *The Monk Who Sold His Ferrari* by Robin Sharma. Patricia designed and is currently leading PsiBeauty, a series of workshops in the field of emotional intelligence, relational health, and sexual education for women. You can visit her website at www.animarom.ro.

PY KIM CONANT: the author of *Sex Secrets of an American Geisha: How to Attract, Satisfy, and Keep Your Man.* You can visit her website at www.AmericanGeishaHouse.com.

LAUREN MICHELLE KUTASI is a Los Angeles native who began her art training as soon as she was able to hold a pencil. During high school she attended the Art Center and eventually graduated college with a BFA. After graduation Lauren's creative skills were put to test as a stylist and costumer, which led her to executive and design positions and eventually publicity. Trained classically and in nontraditional mediums, Lauren has been commissioned to share her artistic ability by means of painting, illustration, fashion, jewelry, and writing. Currently Lauren is focusing on building her name as a writer, artist, and designer. You can visit her website at www.LaurenKutasi.com.

Miss Exotic World 2004, MISS DIRTY MARTINI was named the "Sexpot Sophisticate" by NY Magazine, has been described as "one of the best in burlesque" by the *New York Times*, "the queen of them all" by the *London Telegraph*, and "the decadent expression of female sensuality in action" by the *New York Daily News*. Since the mid 1990s she has been a leading figure in the American burlesque revival and has become an underground celebrity and a favorite of burlesque legends who performed in the 1940s. She has headlined burlesque shows in the United States and in Europe and performed alongside comedian Margaret Cho in her Off-Broadway show The Sensuous Woman. You can visit her website at www.missdirtymartini.com.

ACHSA VISSEL is a Dutch psychologist-sexologist who specializes in teenage problems. She has a private practice in Amsterdam and has written two books including *Vrijen Enzovoort* (Love Making Etc.), a sex education manual for teenagers and Rubenskaarten (Rubenscards), a book to inspire women how to feel good about their bodies. She also has a weekly radio segment on love, sex, and relationships on the largest radio station in Holland and is frequently used as an expert by the Dutch media (newspapers, TV, radio, magazines). You can visit her website at www.achsavissel.nl/achsavissellinks.html.

LISA WIXON was born in the United States in 1969, and grew up in a newspaper family near Lake Tahoe, Nevada. She graduated from the University of Miami with a degree in international and cinema.

Lisa has lived in Europe and Latin America, and has racked up passport stamps from more than forty countries. Her latest stop was Havana, Cuba. Intending to visit for a week, Lisa became captivated with life in Cuba, and stayed nearly a year. She felt compelled to tell the stories of *jineteras* and *jineterors,* the typically educated Cuban doctors, nurses, professors, architects, and students who prostitute themselves to tourists. Her observations and experiences are detailed in the novel Dirty Blonde and Half Cuba (Rayo/Harper Collins). You can visit her website at www.lisawixon.com.

KRISTINA WRIGHT is an award winning author whose erotic fiction has appeared in over sixty anthologies, including *Dirty Girls: Erotica for Women*; *Bedding Down: A Collection of Winter Erotica*; several volumes of *The Mammoth Book of Best New Erotica*; and the nonfiction guide *The Many Joys of Sex Toys*.

Products by Laura Corn

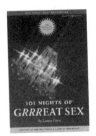

101 Nights of Grrreat Sex
The book that has lit the fire in over two million bedrooms. 101 steamy seductions, written in complete, erotic detail . . . and because they're sealed shut, each one is a delicious secret until you and your lover tear them open and spring your sensuous surprises on each other!

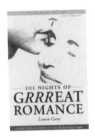

101 Nights Of Grrreat Romance
Not just a romance book—this is real, live romance. Tear open the secret sealed pages and follow Laura's detailed plans for 101 thrilling, romantic adventures. Each one comes as a complete surprise when you and your lover spring them on each other!

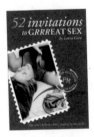

52 Invitations to Grrreat Sex . . . You Won't Believe What's Coming in the Mail!
Once a week—every week for an entire year—Grrreat Sex is in the bag (the mailbag!) Laura has created fifty-two brand-new erotic adventures, each with a unique twist: an invitation, ready to be mailed to your lover. It's steamy but discreet; mysterious, yet perfectly clear. It means a night of heart-pounding, sheet-splitting, toe-curling sex is on the way. . . .

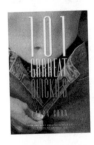

101 Grrreat Quickies
Never again run out of ideas to keep the sizzle in your relationship. The first and only book with 101 Quickie coupons redeemable on the spot for unusual wild sex!

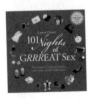

101 Nights of Grrreat Sex: The Game
The Game of Surprises, Sexual Trivia and Secret Sealed Seductions.

Come, flirt, tease, and seduce your lover as you travel around the board on your way to a night of Grrreat Sex.

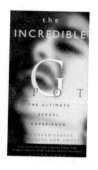

THE INCREDIBLE G-SPOT VIDEO—THE ULTIMATE SEXUAL EXPERIENCE

G-spot Orgasms. Every woman can have one. Every man can give one. It's not a myth!

This video will teach you exactly where the G-spot is, and reveal six advanced sexual techniques for experiencing its pleasures. Sophisticated computer graphics based on actual ultrasonic images of human intercourse, clearly illustrate the best positions for stimulating this extraordinary erogenous zone. Live actors show all six methods in a clear, candid, and highly sensuous demonstration. And the results? Wait until you hear Laura Corn's guests—both men and women—discuss their reaction to discovering the awesome power of the G-spot orgasm for the first time! Must be 21 years of age. Contains full nudity and explicit scenes. 60 minute video.

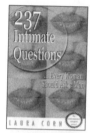

237 INTIMATE QUESTIONS EVERY WOMAN SHOULD ASK A MAN

Laura Corn interviewed 1,000 men to find out what they really think about sex, love, and relationships. These are the questions they most want to be asked by the women in their lives. Plus, mens' outrageous, uncensored answers are sealed up inside.

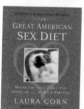

THE GREAT AMERICAN SEX DIET

Two years ago, Laura Corn had a revelation—a new idea that could take couples beyond great sex and great romance. But before she brought it to her fans, she knew she had to put it to the ultimate test.

She secretly gathered thirty-eight couples and asked them to try the plan that would become *The Great American Sex Diet*. What happened next surprised them all.

For twenty-eight amazing, eye-opening days, Laura's volunteers explored the sealed pages in this book and followed Laura's secret recipes. They seduced each other. They surprised each other. They courted each other. And the sex they had was more incredible, wonderful, and breathtaking than they'd had in years. The results were extraordinary. All the successful couples had proven the truth behind Laura Corn's newest insight. Men and women felt better, they listened more, and they treated each other with tenderness and respect. In short, they fell in love all over again.

You'll be inspired by their tales of transformation. And you'll see the results with your own eyes because each intimate story is accompanied by revealing before-and-after portraits that capture the remarkable changes brought on by the diet. *The Great American Sex Diet* can work the same magic in your relationship.

Specialty Shops

FOR CATALOGS INCLUDING many of the products mentioned in this book, contact the following companies.

For Adult Toys, Videos, Books, Massage Oil, etc:

CCYELL
8621–64936311
www.ccyell.com

Good Vibrations
603 Valencia Street
San Francisco, CA 94110
1-800-289-8423
www.goodvibes.com

Love Honey
+0800-915-6635
www.lovehoney.co.uk

My Pleasure
1061 Sneath Lane
San Bruno, CA 94066
1-866-697-5327
www.mypleasure.com

Sexy Wardrobe and Lingerie:

3 Wishes Lingerie, Sexy Costumes and More
2144 East Lyon Station Road
Creedmoor, NC 2752
1-800-438-6605 x 1
www.3wishes.com

Azzuma Fine Imported Lingerie
www.azzuma.com

Cette
+32 (0)53 85 95 30
www.cette.com

Spoylt
+44 115 988-2814
www.spoylt.com

Victoria's Secret
1-800-888-8200
www.victoriassecret.com

Yandy
7801 East Gray Road, Suite 160
Scottsdale, Arizona 85260
1-800-883-0860
www.yandy.com

Laura Corn Products:

www.101nights.com

www.amazon.com

More Grrreat websites:

www.beaumonde.net

www.cosmopolitan.com

www.durex.com

www.gawker.com

www.gridskipper.com

www.ivillage.com

www.jezebel.com

www.madelineinthemirror.com

www.menshealth.com

www.myla.com

www.roadjunky.com

www.scarletmagazine.co.uk

www.tantric.com

www.tinynibbles.com

www.universaltouchinc.com

www.women24.com